ARACHNOID CY

ARACHNOID CYSTS

Epidemiology, Biology, and Neuroimaging

Edited by

KNUT WESTER

University of Bergen, Bergen, Norway
Haukeland University Hospital, Bergen, Norway

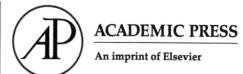

ACADEMIC PRESS

An imprint of Elsevier

Academic Press is an imprint of Elsevier
125 London Wall, London EC2Y 5AS, United Kingdom
525 B Street, Suite 1800, San Diego, CA 92101-4495, United States
50 Hampshire Street, 5th Floor, Cambridge, MA 02139, United States
The Boulevard, Langford Lane, Kidlington, Oxford OX5 1GB, United Kingdom

Notices
Knowledge and best practice in this field are constantly changing. As new research and experience broaden our understanding, changes in research methods, professional practices, or medical treatment may become necessary.

Practitioners and researchers must always rely on their own experience and knowledge in evaluating and using any information, methods, compounds, or experiments described herein. In using such information or methods they should be mindful of their own safety and the safety of others, including parties for whom they have a professional responsibility.

To the fullest extent of the law, neither the Publisher nor the authors, contributors, or editors, assume any liability for any injury and/or damage to persons or property as a matter of products liability, negligence or otherwise, or from any use or operation of any methods, products, instructions, or ideas contained in the material herein.

British Library Cataloguing-in-Publication Data
A catalogue record for this book is available from the British Library

Library of Congress Cataloging-in-Publication Data
A catalog record for this book is available from the Library of Congress

ISBN: 978-0-12-809932-2

For Information on all Academic Press publications
visit our website at https://www.elsevier.com/books-and-journals

Working together
to grow libraries in
developing countries

ELSEVIER Book Aid International

www.elsevier.com • www.bookaid.org

Publisher: Mica Haley
Acquisition Editor: Melanie Tucker
Editorial Project Manager: Kathy Padilla
Production Project Manager: Stalin Viswanathan
Cover Designer: Mark Rogers

Typeset by MPS Limited, Chennai, India

Dedication

To my wife Sidsel for her impatient patience with my mental absence during the last year's work on this project.

Contents

I

INTRODUCTION

1. Arachnoid Cysts—Historical Perspectives and Controversial Aspects
KNUT WESTER

II

BIOLOGICAL ASPECTS

2. Arachnoid Cysts—Intracranial Locations, Gender, and Sidedness
KNUT WESTER

3. Molecular Biology and Genetics: Gene Expression, Twin Studies and Familial Occurrence, and Syndromes Associated With AC
CHRISTIAN A. HELLAND

4. Arachnoid Cysts in Glutaric Aciduria Type I (GA-I)
NIKOLAS BOY AND STEFAN KÖLKER

5. Ultrastructure of Arachnoid Cysts
KATRIN RABIEI AND BENGT R. JOHANSSON

6. Pathophysiology of Intracranial Arachnoid Cysts: Hypoperfusion of Adjacent Cortex
SPYRIDON SGOUROS AND CHRISTOS CHAMILOS

7. Biochemistry—Composition of and Possible Mechanisms for Production of Arachnoid Cyst Fluid
MAGNUS BERLE AND KNUT WESTER

8. The "Valve Mechanism"
DAVID SANTAMARTA AND EMILIO GONZÁLEZ-MARTÍNEZ

III

PREVALENCE AND NATURAL HISTORY OF ARACHNOID CYSTS

9. The Prevalence of Intracranial Arachnoid Cysts
FRANK WEBER

10. Classification and Location of Arachnoid Cysts
CHRISTIAN A. HELLAND

11. Growth and Disappearance of Arachnoid Cysts
KNUT WESTER

12. Arachnoid Cysts and Subdural and Intracystic Hematomas
KNUT WESTER

13. Hydrocephalus Associated With Arachnoid Cysts
JUAN F. MARTÍNEZ-LAGE, CLAUDIO PIQUERAS AND MARÍA-JOSÉ ALMAGRO

IV

NEUROIMAGING

14. Radiological Workup, CT, MRI
JOHAN WIKSTRÖM

15. Arachnoid Cyst—Prenatal Detection, Management, and Perinatal Outcome

BART DE KEERSMAECKER, MICHAEL AERTSEN, LIESBETH THEWISSEN, KATRIEN JANSEN AND LUC DE CATTE

16. SPECT Studies in Patients With Arachnoid Cysts

JUAN F. MARTÍNEZ-LAGE, MARÍA-JOSÉ ALMAGRO AND ANTONIO L. LÓPEZ-GUERRERO

Index 215

List of Contributors

Michael Aertsen UZ Leuven Hospitals, Leuven, Belgium

María-José Almagro Virgen de la Arrixaca University Hospital, Murcia, Spain

Magnus Berle University of Bergen, Bergen, Norway; Haukeland University Hospital, Bergen, Norway

Nikolas Boy University Hospital Heidelberg, Heidelberg, Germany

Christos Chamilos "Mitera" Childrens Hospital, Athens, Greece

Luc De Catte UZ Leuven Hospitals, Leuven, Belgium

Bart De Keersmaecker UZ Leuven Hospitals, Leuven, Belgium; AZ Groeninge Hospital, Kortrijk, Belgium

Emilio González-Martínez University Hospital of León, León, Spain

Christian A. Helland Haukeland University Hospital, Bergen, Norway; University of Bergen, Bergen, Norway

Katrien Jansen UZ Leuven Hospitals, Leuven, Belgium

Bengt R. Johansson University of Gothenburg, Gothenburg, Sweden

Stefan Kölker University Hospital Heidelberg, Heidelberg, Germany

Antonio L. López-Guerrero Virgen de la Arrixaca University Hospital, Murcia, Spain; University of Murcia Medical School, Murcia, Spain

Juan F. Martínez-Lage Virgen de la Arrixaca University Hospital, Murcia, Spain; University of Murcia Medical School, Murcia, Spain

Claudio Piqueras Virgen de la Arrixaca University Hospital, Murcia, Spain; University of Murcia Medical School, Murcia, Spain

Katrin Rabiei Sahlgrenska University Hospital, Gothenburg, Sweden; University of Gothenburg, Gothenburg, Sweden

David Santamarta University Hospital of León, León, Spain

Spyridon Sgouros "Mitera" Childrens Hospital and University of Athens, Athens, Greece

Liesbeth Thewissen UZ Leuven Hospitals, Leuven, Belgium

Frank Weber German Air Force Center of Aerospace Medicine, Fuerstenfeldbruck, Germany

Knut Wester University of Bergen, Bergen, Norway; Haukeland University Hospital, Bergen, Norway

Johan Wikström Uppsala University Hospital, Uppsala, Sweden

Preface

To my knowledge, this is the first textbook in English ever on arachnoid cysts (ACs). Considering the fact that AC is the most common intracranial expansive condition in the general population, this absence of comprehensive literature is striking. Most probably it reflects the common attitude shared by many colleagues: that an AC is a congenital, benign condition that does not require attention unless it yields dramatic symptoms.

More often than for other intracranial conditions, relatively little high level evidence exists on ACs and how we should deal with them. Unfortunately, the majority of publications on the subject are case reports or case series with low levels of evidence and consequently little to build recommendations on. However, there are also studies that have investigated AC related matters in larger cohorts and in a systematic fashion. In this book, emphasis is placed on such extensive and systematic reports when they exist, rather than on reports describing a few patients.

However, if a large collection of case reports point in the same direction, such evidence cannot be completely dismissed. Less weight must be put on "experts' opinions" if they are based only on clinical experience achieved back in the time when any intracranial procedure was a risky undertaking, attitudes that have been conveyed to us from previous generations of colleagues without any questioning of the truth of the message in the meantime. It is my impression, after having read hundreds of publications in preparing this book, that this lack of systematically collected evidence in the past has allowed mindsets acquired decades ago to survive and maintain the status of truth, even if the basis of this "wisdom" is very weak, see e.g., Chapter 1, Arachnoid Cysts—Historical Perspectives and Controversial Aspects, in this volume.

In an attempt to sort out what is the truth and what are myths and misconceptions (or whatever lies inbetween), we have asked a total of 43 international colleagues from 10 different countries on three continents, with views that we knew or assumed to be conflicting, to contribute to the chapters in this book. Some of these authors have vast clinical and scientific experience with the topic; others are less merited, but nevertheless have an interesting story to tell. The authors were asked to base their chapters on existing evidence and to indicate the evidence levels for their statements in the beginning of each chapter when possible. Otherwise they were given free hands, thus allowing opposing views to be exposed.

This liberal editorial attitude may well have resulted in conflicting or even confusing information, but so are the views and opinions of our colleagues; it is therefore of importance that they all are represented here in this book. Thus, my advice to the readers is simply to read and evaluate the conflicting evidence and in the end: make up your own minds—to do the best for our patients.

Due to the amount of available information, this textbook is published in two separate volumes. As the subtitle indicates, the present volume (Volume 1—Epidemiology, Biology, and Neuroimaging) gives information about aspects that are not directly related to clinical practice, with the exception of the last three chapters (14–16) that are focused on neuroimaging diagnostics. In addition, Chapter 1, Arachnoid Cysts—Historical Perspectives and Controversial Aspects, attempts to provide the reader with historical information that may be of help in understanding some of the present-day views on ACs.

Guy Eslick, Professor of Cancer Epidemiology and Medical Statistics at The University of Sydney, Australia took the initiative for the book by suggesting that I write and edit a book on this topic. Without this initiative, for which I am very grateful, this book would never have materialized.

I would also like to express my gratitude to the editorial staff at Elsevier: Kathy Padilla and Melanie Tucker for their friendly and expeditious advice and assistance.

Knut Wester

PART I

INTRODUCTION

Arachnoid Cysts—Historical Perspectives and Controversial Aspects

Knut Wester[1,2]

[1]University of Bergen, Bergen, Norway
[2]Haukeland University Hospital, Bergen, Norway

O U T L I N E

Arachnoid Cysts: Epidemiology, Biology, and Neuroimaging
DOI: http://dx.doi.org/10.1016/B978-0-12-809932-2.00001-6

ABBREVIATIONS

AC   arachnoid cyst
CNS   central nervous system
CT   computerized tomography
MRI   magnetic resonance imaging

Everything has its history, as do arachnoid cysts (ACs), although it may be difficult to trace it in the literature, as the name of the condition has changed over time. For instance, one of the earliest scientific reports on the condition [1], referred to it as "chronic cystic arachnoiditis"; before that, Horrax published an article on "cisternal arachnoiditis" [2]. Other names that were used during the early years were "pia-AC" and "meningitis serosa."

THE EARLY HISTORY

The First Observation and Description of an AC

The English physician Richard Bright (1789–1858) (Fig. 1.1) served most of his time at Guy's Hospital in London together with other renowned physicians, such as Thomas Addison and Thomas Hodgkin.

He is regarded by many as the father of nephrology, and has a disease named after him in that field of medicine: Bright's disease. He had,

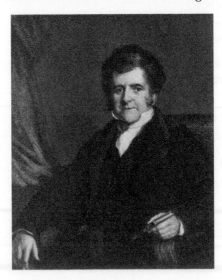

FIGURE 1.1   Portrait of Richard Bright (1789–1858), English physician. *Source: From Thomas Joseph Pettigrew, Medical Portrait Gallery vol. 2 (1838).*

however, a much broader interest in medicine than only kidney diseases. At Guy's Hospital, Bright soon appreciated the importance of autopsies in the understanding of diseases and combined this interest with his gifts as an artist to draw and paint both normal and diseased organs. Based on the combinations of these two interests, he published a large book on morbid anatomy in at least two large volumes: "Reports of Medical Cases, Selected with a View of Illustrating the Symptoms and Cure of Diseases by a Reference to Morbid Anatomy." Volume II "Diseases of the Brain and Nervous System − Part I" alone constitutes 450 pages of text in addition to 14 full page plates with detailed paintings of the affected organs [3].

In this volume, he described two cases of cysts in the arachnoid, both found at autopsy. Figure 1 on Plate II in this volume is probably the first depiction of an AC in the literature (Fig. 1.2).

Bright did not only look superficially at this case, he gave a very thorough account of the case story and the autopsy finding on pages 437−439, as will be apparent from below.

First he gives an accurate description and interpretation of these cysts that he, with a high degree of precision, called "Serous Cysts in the Arachnoid." In these few pages (437−439) he wrote about the subject, based on the autopsy finding in only two patients—he apparently had grasped the true nature of these cysts; in the following quotations, I have underlined those passages of his description and interpretations that still are valid:

> There is a species of partial accumulation of fluid in the brain, which must not be passed over without notice: I mean, serous cysts forming in connection with the

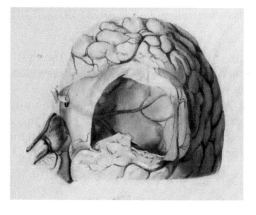

FIGURE 1.2 The first depiction of an AC, illustrated by Richard Bright. *Source: From "Reports of Medical Cases, Selected with a View of Illustrating the Symptoms and Cure of Diseases by a Reference to Morbid Anatomy." Volume II "Diseases of the Brain and Nervous System − Part I": Figure 1 on plate II [3].*

arachnoid, and apparently lying between its layers, or attached by thin adventitious membranes. These are occasionally discovered on dissection; and have either produced no symptoms, or have been quite unsuspected till after death. These cysts vary from the size of a pea to that of a large orange, and may be considerably larger. They appear to be of the most chronic character, and probably never enlarge after their first formation. The brain is completely impressed by them, so that when the fluid is let out, a permanent cavity remains, and even the bone of the skull is moulded to their form. I have given the representation of these cysts, as they occurred in two cases, in Plate XXI. Fig. 4. and Plate II. Fig. 1.

Then he went on to describe the case depicted in Plate II Fig. 1.1. in more detail, including the autopsy report—the illness that killed the poor tailor probably had no correlation to the unexpected autopsy finding of a large cyst; he probably died of a "fever." Thus, the cyst can probably be regarded as an incidental finding:

> CASE XXVI. — William Tennant, aetat. 18, (tailor,) admitted on the 14th Jan. 1829, had been unwell with the usual symptoms of fever for eight days; no treatment had been adopted. He complained, on admission, of epigastric tenderness; slight headach;...
>
> 17. (January) Pain of forehead gone; less flushing; tendency to coma, and rambling, from which he is easily aroused, and answers intelligibly when questioned. Cont. med.
>
> 18. Pulse 112; passed a restless night, without sleep, but was more delirious; sensible, at present, but lapses frequently into a muttering dose; ...
>
> 21. Died last evening. Dissection.—On sawing through the skull cap, a sudden gush of limpid fluid attracted attention; and on carefully removing it, and examining whence this fluid escaped, a considerable oblong depression was found in the middle lobe of the right hemisphere. On minute inspection, the fluid, which amounted to at least twelve ounces, had been contained in a cyst formed by the splitting of the arachnoid membrane, which had pressed on the middle lobe of the brain, and thus produced a corresponding depression. The membranes and substance of the brain, (with the exception stated,) did not exhibit any morbid appearances.

Bright's accurate observation in 1829, that the cyst was formed by splitting of the arachnoid, precedes the next observation (in 1958) of the same by Starkman et al. [4] by nearly 130 years.

When reading old articles from before the computed tomography (CT) era, the distribution of cyst locations is strikingly different from what we see today. Rengachary and Watanabe [5] performed a survey of the literature and found a total of 208 cysts.

Where Were the Early Cysts Located?

In 1924, Horrax published a large series of patients with "Generalized cisternal arachnoiditis simulating cerebellar tumor" in the posterior fossa, all operated in ether narcosis at Peter Bent Brigham

Hospital during the period 1913–22, mostly by Harvey Cushing, but also by Horrax himself [2]. After having read this extensively detailed report, including description of the surgical procedures, it becomes clear that at least 28 of these cases most probably had an AC in the posterior fossa. Preoperatively, most of the patients displayed cerebellar symptoms and impaired vision due to secondary hydrocephalus. Three patients died in the immediate postoperative phase, and two patients died after a follow-up period of 2 years, presumably of unrelated causes. The surviving 23 patients were observed for 1–9 years; 12 were then without complaints, classified as "well," the remaining 11 were "improved." This improvement applies also to the reduced vision in most of the patients.

In 1962 Lewis presented a survey of the literature, ranging 30 years back to 1932 [6]. He mentioned, but did not include those cases presented by Horrax in 1924. Lewis noted that "Cases of arachnoid cyst or cystic arachnoiditis reported in the literature appear to fall into three pathological categories." One type was believed to be of inflammatory origin, the other group was "made up of cysts following fractures of the parietal region with unhealed dural tears with skull fracture." The 27 cysts in the third group, which Lewis called "sporadic," had no obvious cause as they were "not associated with arachnoid adhesions or with gross pathological evidence of trauma." It is not possible to retrieve sufficient information from these early publications included in the survey to decide the exact nature of these "sporadic" cysts, but one gets the impression that most of them probably were ACs as we know them today. As many as 18 of these 27 cysts retrieved by Lewis were located in the posterior fossa, e.g., the one described by Craig [1] (Fig. 1.3), the remaining nine "were above the tentorium, in or near the Sylvian fissure."

R.G. Robinson of New Zealand concentrated on "Intracranial collections of fluid with local bulging of the skull" and published a total of seven cases of cysts in the middle fossa [7,8]. He also reviewed the literature and found at least nine more similar cases, as presented in his Table 1 [7]. Unfortunately, he later coined this condition temporal lobe agenesis, although the term "arachnoid cyst" already was well established, see below.

As methods for literature search were rather deficient in 1962, a Web of Science search was performed for the present chapter, searching for "arachnoid cyst OR cystic arachnoiditis OR pia-AC OR Meningitis Serosa," all terms that had been used for ACs since the beginning of the 20th century. Not all titles were available for reading, but it was possible to retrieve a total of 10 publications in the 30 years following the publication of Craig [1]; most of them were already included in Lewis' survey. The search revealed another 11 cysts that were not included in

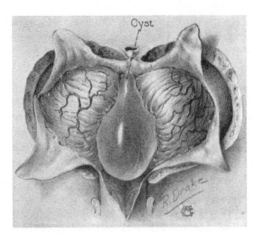

FIGURE 1.3   Cyst in the posterior fossa as published by Craig. *Source: Reprinted from Craig, W. McK. (1932). Chronic cystic arachnoiditis. Am J Surg 17, 384–388 [1].*

the publications of Robinson and Lewis; they were all located in the posterior fossa [1,9–11].

Thus, at least 82 ACs were published in the period 1932–1962, 57 in the posterior fossa, and 25 above the tentorium. This distribution of cysts, with a large majority being located in the posterior fossa, seems to be in striking contrast to the distribution we know today. In the only population-based study, including a total of 299 patients, only 12% of them had posterior fossa cysts; the vast majority were found above the tentorium [12].

So, one may wonder: why this difference in cyst location between the early years and now? It seems reasonable to assume that it has something to do with the near-complete lack of radiological imaging, leaving the diagnosis more or less to clinical observations, favoring cysts located in small intracranial compartments with important content. The small volume of the posterior fossa does not allow much extra volume, e.g., a cyst, before the pressure increases to abnormal values, affecting the nervous structures there. Some of these are of vital importance, such as the brainstem, whereas the cerebellum or the cranial nerves may rapidly give distinct, neurological focal deficits. Another important symptom in the reports from those early years was reduced vision, as a consequence of a longstanding, secondary hydrocephalus. Contrary to the posterior fossa, the much larger supratentorial compartment allows an extra volume more easily and areas that may yield focal neurological deficits are more widespread than in the densely packed posterior fossa. Thus, in the early days of neurosurgery, cysts in the posterior fossa had a much higher chance of being discovered than supratentorial cysts; a high proportion of the latter were discovered because of asymmetry—"bulging"—of the skull and radiological thinning of the bone and not all were operated [7,8].

ARACHNOID CYSTS AND IMAGING

Skull X-Ray and Angiograms

The visualization of the central nervous system (CNS) is hampered by the fact that CNS is enclosed in tissue (bone) with a much higher radiodensity than the brain or the spinal cord, thus leaving these structures inaccessible for plain X-ray diagnostics, with a very few exceptions. R.G. Robinson used bulging and thinning of the temporal bone overlying an AC ("temporal lobe agenesis") as a radiological indication in addition to an enlarged middle fossa and a raised sphenoid wing. Later, invasive techniques were used to give indirect evidence of an expansion, above all the steep course of sphenoid wing (Fig. 1.4) and

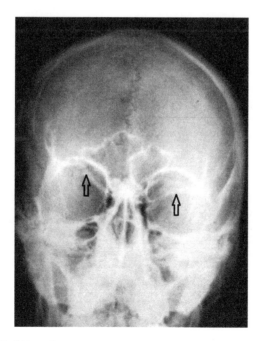

FIGURE 1.4   Skull X-ray demonstrating a very steep course of the right sphenoid wing compared with the normal course (arrows) on the left side. *Source: Reprinted from Robinson, R.G. Temporal lobe agenesis syndrome. 1964. Brain, 87, 87–106. [13] by permission of Oxford University Press.*

the carotid and middle cerebral arteries on the affected side. Angiography was a relatively dangerous procedure at that time, as it required puncture and direct contrast injection into the carotid artery of the neck.

The CT Era

It was not until the integration of radiological and computer techniques that it was possible to depict CNS tissue directly, as this development made it possible to bypass the hindrance of the radiopaque bone of the skull and spine. The English engineer Godfrey Newbold Hounsfield (1919–2004 Fig. 1.5) was instrumental in developing the revolutionary, new technique of CT, for which he was awarded the Nobel Prize for Physiology or Medicine in 1979. Fig. 1.6 shows the first CT scanner, the EMI scanner from 1970 to 1971, produced by the British music record company EMI.

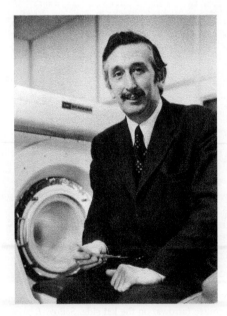

FIGURE 1.5   The engineer behind the development of the first CT scanner, Sir Godfrey Newbold Hounsfield. *Source: Photo by Central Press/Hulton Archive/Getty Images.*

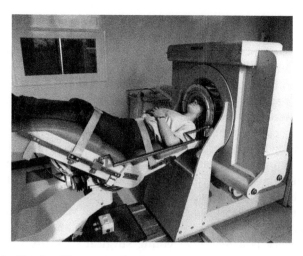

FIGURE 1.6   The first CT scanner, the EMI CT brain scanner-1970–71.

ARACHNOID CYSTS: CONTROVERSIES AND MISCONCEPTIONS

The Reluctance to Operate ACs—Can It Be Explained From the History?

There (still) seems to exist a surprisingly marked reluctance to operate intracranial ACs, even when the patients harboring such cysts have marked symptoms, such as headache, vertigo/dizziness, or epilepsy; symptoms that we usually accept as most likely being caused by intracranial expansive processes of a different nature, e.g., neoplasms. As will be discussed below, I believe this reluctance may be based on outdated views and misconceptions about ACs that possibly can be understood if we go back in time and look at them in a historical perspective. To do this, we have to look at a combination of how neurosurgery has developed and the methods by which neurosurgical residents are trained.

Surgery was not a medical discipline until it was incorporated into classical medicine in the decades around 1800; it was not until the end of the Age of Enlightenment that the medical profession recognized the value of surgery, and included the trade as a formal discipline. Before that time, surgeons were craftsmen, trained first as apprentices by a master of the trade, sometimes in *surgical academies*, but never inside universities. Not until the medical profession saw the advantages of such procedures, was surgery invited in and taken up by the classical medicine that had existed for centuries. Still, surgery is very much a handicraft, naturally, in which you learn the trade from your more experienced seniors, the masters. In that setting, the master possesses the wisdom and knows the tricks of the trade, which is passed on to the apprentices, often in a practical nonscholarly fashion. Even today, surgical training requires both an academic education as well as development of the necessary trade skills.

Thus, surgical disciplines, neurosurgery included, have a double background, both as an academic discipline and as a trade. In the latter tradition, it is a good idea to listen to and adopt what the seniors teach. In the former, one can move the discipline forward by questioning and examining the validity of old truths. When going back in time, the AC does not seem to have evoked any great interest, as reflected in the scientific literature.

Neurosurgery is a relatively young surgical specialty that has gone through a fantastic development over the last 5–6 decades. However, back in the 1950s intracranial surgery was still a dangerous undertaking with high morbidity and mortality. At that time, the old masters of the trade wisely admonished their apprentices never to operate on such benign intracranial cysts, as a craniotomy was a risky procedure, especially when the indication was not to save lives, but rather to improve the quality of life. When these early apprentices later became "masters of the trade" themselves, they conceivably continued to convey this supposed wisdom to their apprentices without questioning the underlying truth. Thus, by passing on this "common knowledge" to their own novices, they further cemented the myth.

I believe this preserved transfer of old knowledge from masters to apprentices without a willingness to examine its validity is one important reason for all the misunderstandings associated with ACs. It was good advice when the master of the trade at that time said: "Don't ever operate benign intracranial cysts," as the procedure was much too risky for a procedure aimed at improving quality of life. Other words of wisdom that I was taught myself during my residency, were that the patients' symptoms had nothing to do with the cyst and that a surgical decompression would not relieve the patients' complaints, an assumption that is not supported by research or personal experience, as will be apparent from this book.

The introduction of an awkward new name for the condition, "temporal lobe agenesis" in the 1950s [7,8], *further added to the confusion*—as it implied that the condition was not an expansive cyst, but an underdeveloped temporal lobe, with the vacant temporal fossa somehow filled up by CSF instead of brain tissue.

The Big Mistake—The Temporal Lobe Agenesis Syndrome

In 1955, the New Zealand neurosurgeon Richard G. Robinson questioned the cystic nature of the fluid collection in the temporal fossa that he had observed in patients with a bulging and thinning of the overlying skull bone [7]. When discussing this phenomenon, he wrote: "It is suggested that this condition of a fluid collection in the region usually occupied by the temporal pole of the brain and associated with enlargement of the boundaries of the middle cranial fossa is caused primarily by agenesis of the temporal lobe."

At 40 days' gestation, the cerebral hemisphere has the shape of a ball, but soon after it starts to curve around what will be the Sylvian fissure. During this curving, the posterior, inferior part of this early ball-shaped hemispheric anlage moves forward and develops into the temporal lobe. Robinson attributed the lack of the temporal lobe to a failure of this process.

He had, however, problems explaining how the lack of brain tissue could lead to the increased volume of the temporal fossa that he too had observed in these cases: "It is less easy to account for the expansion of the skull. It is well known that most types of agenesis of the brain are associated with a corresponding lack of development of the skull on that side."

His attempts at explaining this apparent self-contradiction are however, far from clear and convincing: "Pascal's law states that in a fluid, the pressure applied at any point is transmitted equally in all directions. Yet with these pathological conditions there is some local escape from this law. Connolly has suggested that the digital impressions of the skull in adolescence and in hydrocephalic states result from a closer contact of the brain surface with the inner table of the skull than previously. Close tissue proximity certainly occurs with most hematomas and tumours, and produces, perhaps, what are no more than gigantic digital impressions. Somehow or other the fluid collections in temporal lobe agenesis act similarly although the dynamic factors are far from clear."

His theory met some opposition, and in 1958 he went on with his attempts at finding an explanation to defend his model: "It is contended that the primary defect of the syndrome is the agenesis. .... Many operative accounts have indicated that the brain was compressed and dislocated by cysts which might contain up to 500 c.c. of fluid. .... It is unlikely that any such displacement of the brain would be compatible with life, let alone any lack of gross neurological disturbance. It is suggested that in fact parts of the brain were absent and their site was occupied by an external hydrocephalus" [8].

Six years later, Robinson continued elaborating on his ideas and attacking his opponents, first and foremost Starkman et al., who had insisted that these were true cysts: "It is, however, difficult to account for the expansion of the skull unless the fluid was encysted and behaved as an expanding mass" [4]. Without any further convincing arguments, Robinson then stated that: "We can see no reason to alter our contention that the fluid collection is a true external hydrocephalus and not a cyst," and "'The temporal lobe agenesis syndrome' is suggested to cover this entity which would include many cases previously described as chronic subdural hygroma or hydroma, and arachnoid cysts and its synonyms" [13].

If the primary event was an underdeveloped temporal lobe, there would of course be no indication for a decompressing procedure. Therefore, surgical decompressions were brought to a halt as a consequence of the widely accepted belief in the "temporal lobe agenesis" hypothesis.

At last, Robinson publicly denounced his earlier view that agenesis of the temporal lobe was the primary, underlying event behind these cysts. In a strong and frank statement in 1971, he agreed with his previous opponents, whom he gave full credit in this most admirable way: "Robinson (1964) coined the phrase 'temporal lobe agenesis' to describe the middle fossa lesions. This title should be abandoned and the syndrome takes its place amongst the other arachnoid malformations. The account of Starkman, Brown and Linell (1958) is a landmark in the modern literature on arachnoid cysts" [14]. Such honesty is rare to find in science; one could only wish for it to occur more often.

Nevertheless, the idea of a temporal lobe agenesis syndrome appears to have had a life of its own for many years after that, even if it was no longer supported by its father. One example is the article by Robertson et al., where the authors seem to accept the notion of a primary agenesis or hypogenesis: "We would add that if the MR study demonstrates hypogenesis of the temporal lobe without compression, or if the compression is mild and not causing elevated intracranial pressure, surgery is not indicated" [15]. The concept of the temporal lobe agenesis also had a long life outside the neurosurgical literature; I have myself seen an AC described as "temporal lobe agenesis" by an experienced neuroradiologist in the late 1990s.

Other Misconceptions

"ACs are just incidental findings without functional significance." This may be true for those cysts that are found when reviewing brain CTs or MRIs from large populations, especially in populations that were scanned for other reasons than clinical symptoms, such as scanning potential pilots for possible intracranial pathology [16]. Most often a head scan is not requested without a reason, it is prompted by clinical symptoms, most often headache, but also dizziness or epilepsy; an AC disclosed on this background can hardly be classified as "incidental." Some other, rather common misconceptions are all related to the pre- or postoperative cyst volume, such as "small cysts don't give symptoms," as opposed to larger cysts. Another is the belief that a "reduced cyst volume is a prerequisite for clinical improvement." Systematic studies have failed to support these two assumptions, which until recently have been widely accepted as "common knowledge" in the neurological and neurosurgical community. The cyst size does not seem to correlate with symptom intensity [17], but the intracystic *pressure* matters [18]. Postoperative volume reduction is not correlated with clinical improvement in adults [19], whereas such a correlation appears to exist in children [20].

Many of the topics discussed above will be dealt with in more detail in the following chapters.

References

[1] Craig WM. Chronic cystic arachnoiditis. American Journal of Surgery 1932;17:384–8.

[2] Horrax G. Generalized cisternal arachnoiditis simulating cerebellar tumor: its surgical treatment and end-results, 9. Chicago: Archives of Surgery; 1924. p. 95–112.

[3] Bright, R. Serous Cysts in the Arachnoid Diseases of the Brain and Nervous System. In: Reports of Medical Cases Selected With a View of Illustrating the Symptoms and Cure of Diseases by a Reference to Morbid Anatomy. Part I; Vol 2. 1831, London: Longman, Rees, Orme, Brown, and Green.

[4] Starkman SP, Brown TC, Linell EA. Cerebral arachnoid cysts. J Neuropathol Exp Neurol 1958;17(3):484–500.

[5] Rengachary SS, Watanabe I. Ultrastructure and pathogenesis of intracranial arachnoid cysts. J Neuropathol Exp Neurol 1981;40(1):61–83.

[6] Lewis AJ. Infantile hydrocephalus caused by arachnoid cyst. Case report. J Neurosurg 1962;19:431–4.

[7] Robinson RG. Intracranial collections of fluid with local bulging of the skull. J Neurosurg 1955;12(4):345–53.

[8] Robinson RG. Local bulging of the skull and external hydrocephalus due to cerebral agenesis. Br J Radiol 1958;31(372):691–700.

[9] Gardner WJ, Abdullah AF, Mc CL. The varying expressions of embryonal atresia of the fourth ventricle in adults: Arnold-Chiari malformation, Dandy-Walker syndrome, arachnoid cyst of the cerebellum, and syringomyelia. J Neurosurg 1957;14(6):591–605.

[10] Gardner WJ, Mc CL, Dohn DF. Embryonal atresia of the fourth ventricle. The cause of "arachnoid cyst" of the cerebellopontine angle. J Neurosurg 1960;17:226–37.

[11] Lourie H, Berne AS. Radiological and clinical features of an arachnoid cyst of the quadrigeminal cistern. J Neurol Neurosurg Psychiatry 1961;24:374–8.

[12] Helland CA, Lund-Johansen M, Wester K. Location, sidedness, and sex distribution of intracranial arachnoid cysts in a population-based sample. J Neurosurg 2010;113(5): 934–9.

[13] Robinson RG. The Temporal Lobe Agenesis Syndrome. Brain 1964;87:87–106.

[14] Robinson RG. Congenital cysts of the brain: arachnoid malformation. Prog Neurol Surg 1971;4:133–74.

[15] Robertson SJ, Wolpert SM, Runge VM. MR imaging of middle cranial fossa arachnoid cysts: temporal lobe agenesis syndrome revisited. AJNR Am J Neuroradiol 1989;10(5): 1007–10.

[16] Weber F, Knopf H. Incidental findings in magnetic resonance imaging of the brains of healthy young men. J Neurol Sci 2006;240(1–2):81–4.

[17] Morkve SH, et al. Surgical decompression of arachnoid cysts leads to improved quality of life: a prospective study. Neurosurgery 2016;78:613.

[18] Helland CA, Wester K. Intracystic pressure in patients with temporal arachnoid cysts: a prospective study of preoperative complaints and postoperative outcome. J Neurol Neurosurg Psychiatry 2007;78(6):620–3.

[19] Helland CA, Wester K. A population based study of intracranial arachnoid cysts: clinical and neuroimaging outcomes following surgical cyst decompression in adults. J Neurol Neurosurg Psychiatry 2007;78(10):1129–35.

[20] Helland CA, Wester K. A population-based study of intracranial arachnoid cysts: clinical and neuroimaging outcomes following surgical cyst decompression in children. J Neurosurg 2006;105(Suppl. 5):385–90.

PART II

BIOLOGICAL ASPECTS

Arachnoid Cysts—Intracranial Locations, Gender, and Sidedness

Knut Wester[1,2]

[1]University of Bergen, Bergen, Norway [2]Haukeland University Hospital, Bergen, Norway

ABBREVIATIONS

CPA cerebellopontine angle
CT computerized tomography
MRI magnetic resonance imaging

Arachnoid Cysts: Epidemiology, Biology, and Neuroimaging
DOI: http://dx.doi.org/10.1016/B978-0-12-809932-2.00002-8

INTRODUCTION

Arachnoid cysts (AC) are apparently not distributed at random within the neurocranium. Many authors have reported the special affinity for the middle cranial fossa [1–6], with more temporal cysts being located in the left temporal fossa than in the right, and with male preponderance [4–8]. All these publications report results from hospital-based populations with symptomatic ACs; most of the included cysts have therefore caused strong enough complaints to precipitate a neuroimaging examination. It is therefore conceivable that the observed gender and anatomical distribution in the past does not reflect the true distribution in the population and that there somehow has been a selection bias.

From the early 1970s, the threshold for requiring a neuroradiological investigation has gradually been lowered as computed tomography replaced invasive and potentially dangerous diagnostic procedures, but mainly as a consequence of the quantitative explosion of this technology (computerized tomography (CT) and MRI) throughout the world during the last decades. In 1981, Rengachary and Watanabe [9] were the first to compile patient data from previous publications on the distribution of intracranial AC. In their literature search, they found that nearly half (49%) of all intracranial AC were located in the middle fossa. This review, however, included publications that primarily were based on patients diagnosed at autopsy or before the era of CT, when the diagnostic workup included invasive radiological methods, such as cerebral angiography with direct puncture of the carotid arteries, and may therefore not be representative. It is conceivable that patients with severe symptoms were overrepresented in their study, which again may have biased the observed distribution of both intracranial location and sidedness of the cysts. Similarly, it could be that symptoms from the speech dominant hemisphere in these earlier days were given a greater significance as justification for invasive radiological procedures, and that this may be the explanation of the observed left hemisphere preponderance.

In any case, one would expect the widespread application of computed imaging to increase the detection rate of AC, especially the clinically silent ones, and a more correct panorama to emerge, as our group once demonstrated that the apparent left-sidedness of intracerebral benign cysts no longer could be detected when we included in our survey only cases that had been diagnosed after the introduction of computed imaging [10].

To minimize bias related to patient selection for neuroimaging investigations, the present author therefore conducted a literature search for articles published during the last third of the CT era, when computed imaging had become more available than it had been before [4]. For this survey, reports on the occurrence of AC published in the period covered by Index Medicus 1986–90 were surveyed with respect to information about gender of the patients and side of the lesion. Only cases with middle fossa cysts were included. A total of 148 published patients with AC were included, of these 110 were males and 38 were females, giving a male/female ratio of 2.9:1.0 for temporal cysts. There were significantly more lesions in the left middle fossa than on the other side, with a left-to-right ratio of 1.8:1.0.

Thus, after computed imaging had been available for a couple of decades, middle fossa ACs still seemed to occur more frequently on the left side, and more frequently in males than in females in hospital-based populations. However, completely asymptomatic cysts may still exist that would have escaped detection as there was no clinical indication for computed imaging. Therefore, to verify or eventually rule out that the observed sidedness is real, other types of studies were needed, studies that investigated the occurrence of ACs in very large "normal" populations. Such data are now available in four studies [2,3,7,8]; they report on true incidental findings in large populations of healthy individuals. They confirm at least the predilection for the temporal fossa and the left-sidedness and male preponderance of temporal cysts, with 70%–73% of incidentally found cysts being located in the temporal fossa with a left-to right ratio for unilateral temporal cysts being somewhere between 2:1 and 3:1.

Thus, it seems highly unlikely that the observed anatomical distribution in hospital-based populations is caused by a biased selection; one can assume that the predilection for the temporal fossae and the left-sidedness and male dominance of these cysts in fact reflect a true biological phenomenon. Based on this reassuring knowledge, we can go back to reports that describe large series of AC patients to extract more details, preferably recent ones, to benefit from the increased availability of computed imaging.

ANATOMICAL LOCATION, SIDEDNESS, AND GENDER DISTRIBUTION IN LARGE SERIES OF AC PATIENTS

The data presented here are consequently extracted from hospital-based studies published during the last 15 years that comprise at least 30 patients [7,8,11–20]. Some of these give full information about anatomical distribution, sidedness, and gender preponderance, others only information about some of these aspects.

Anatomical Location of ACs

In the following, we will deal specifically with the middle intracranial fossa and the cerebellopontine angle (CPA), since the positioning of an AC in these locations appears to be governed by some biological laws rather than by chance.

In a large hospital-based study from a well-defined geographical area with a stable population, 299 patients with 305 ACs were studied with respect to the aspects discussed here [5]. We will use this report to indicate a rough estimate of the anatomical and gender distribution, as they seem to be fairly representative of what is found in the other publications included in this survey.

The anatomical distribution in this patient series was as follows: middle intracranial fossa 66.9%; frontal convexity 13.8%; posterior fossa 11.8%; and other locations 7.5%. There was a significant sidedness in two locations only; for unilateral cysts in the temporal fossa (six patients had bitemporal cysts) a *left*-sidedness with a left-to-right ratio of 2.5:1.0. Contrary to the temporal fossa, there was a significant and very marked *right*-sidedness for cysts in CPA with 14 on the right and only two on the left side, giving a right-to-left ratio of 7:1. There was no sidedness for any other location. These were the only two locations that also showed significant gender preponderance with a male-to-female ratio of 2.1:1.0 for the temporal cysts and a significant female preponderance for CPA cysts with a female-to-male ratio of 2.2:1.0. As for sidedness, the other locations did not exhibit any gender preponderance.

To sum up the results of this study: AC have a strong predilection for the temporal fossa; there appears to be gender dependency for temporal cysts and cysts in CPA; and cysts in these two locations also exhibit a significant sidedness.

The *predilection for the temporal fossa* varies considerably between the publications included in this review; many report percentages ranging from 63 to 80 [5,13,14,16,18], some report figures in the 40s and 50s [7,8,19,20] and in a few, the figures are so low—in the low—30s—that there hardly seems to be any predilection for the middle fossa at all [12,15,17]. However, as the number of included AC patients also varies considerably between the publications—from 32 to 488—and all the publications indicating low frequencies for temporal cysts comprise few patients, it might be an idea to perform a pooled analysis of all the patients that have been reported in the included studies. That will probably give a better estimate of how often ACs are located in the middle fossa. Doing so, we found 1108 patients with temporal cysts in a total population of 1813 AC patients. Thus, in all AC patients published in the included series above, *temporal cysts comprise 61.1% of all intracranial cysts* (Fig. 2.1).

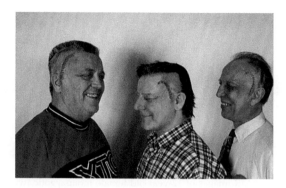

FIGURE 2.1   Three male patients with a temporal AC operated during the same week, illustrating the male preponderance and left-sidedness (two left, one right) for temporal fossa cysts. *Source: Published with permission of the depicted persons.*

Sidedness and Gender

It is however difficult to analyze and calculate figures for *temporal cyst sidedness* in a similar manner because such information is missing in most of the included series [5,7,8,13,14] and because the by far largest series [14] reports an extremely skewed left/right distribution, 222 and 36, respectively. If this report is included in the pooled analysis, the left-to-right ratio for temporal cysts is 646:220 = 3.0:1.0; if it is left out, the left-to-right ratio is 424:184 = 2.3:1.0.

The male/female ratio for any of the other cyst locations is even more difficult to calculate, because so few of the reports give this information [5,15,17,20]. An account of the gender distribution for temporal cysts was given for only 288 patients—190 of them in males and 98 in females—giving a male-to-female ratio of 1.9:1.0.

CPA is the only other intracranial cyst location that appears to exhibit sidedness and gender preponderance, although opposite to those of the temporal fossa, with a female preponderance and right-sidedness. The available information regarding this site is also scarce; only five articles give some information on CPA cysts [5,7,8,11,20]. As mentioned above, there is a strong female preponderance for this location; all the publications that give information on gender report this phenomenon [5,11,20]. A pooled analysis of the available information shows that there were 24 females and only seven males with a CPA cyst, giving a female-to-male ratio of 3.4:1.0. In addition to these three studies, Al-Holou et al. also report a statistically significant right female preponderance [7], however, without giving exact details. The right-sidedness for CPA is also reported by all three articles [5,7,8], although with a varying degree of sidedness; a pooled analysis gives a right-to-left ratio of 1.8. In two of these studies [5,7], the right-sidedness was highly significant.

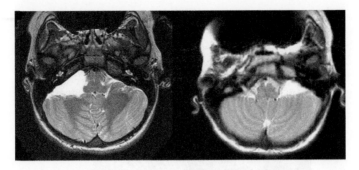

FIGURE 2.2   Axial MR images of 12-year-old female monozygotic twins. Left: the twin with a symptomatic arachnoid cyst in the right cerebellopontine angle (CPA). She suffered from invalidating headache after a minor head injury whilst playing soccer. Right: the asymptomatic sister with a mirror image arachnoid cyst in the left CPA [21].

DISCUSSION

It is conceivable that patients with severe symptoms were overrepresented in earlier hospital-based studies on intracranial AC location or sidedness, which again may have biased the observed and reported distribution. However, information from very large series of "normal" individuals is now available [2,3,7,8]; these studies leave no doubt about the validity of the observed predilection for the temporal fossa, as well as the left-sidedness and male preponderance for temporal cysts. Consequently, one can rule out the possibility of a selection bias caused by symptom severity; these peculiarities must have a biological explanation. Large, hospital-based studies from the last 15 years, when computed tomography has been easily available, add to this information. In addition, some of these recent hospital-based studies give interesting observations on CPA cysts, which also appear to be associated with a gender preponderance and sidedness, except that for the CPA cysts the gender preponderance is female [5,11,20] and the sidedness is right [5,7,8]!

The question of whether a pathological condition has an intracranial predilection site or occurs more frequently in either of the two sexes or on either of the two sides of the body, may seem rather trivial. However, such observations may carry information of some importance for the understanding of that phenomenon and its etiology. It is reasonable to assume a biological mechanism behind the gender preponderance and sidedness, whatever that mechanism might be. Observations of ACs in monozygotic twins [21], in association with other hereditary conditions [22] and their occurrence in families [23,24], as well as certain genetic aspects of the AC membrane [25,26] all suggest that genetic mechanisms somehow are involved in the formation and distribution of such cysts. How these genetic factors, however, can precipitate the formation of an AC eludes me!

References

[1] Arai H, et al. Arachnoid cysts of the middle cranial fossa: experience with 77 patients who were treated with cystoperitoneal shunting. Neurosurgery 1996;39(6):1108–12, discussion 1112-3.

[2] Vernooij MW, et al. Incidental findings on brain MRI in the general population. N Engl J Med 2007;357(18):1821–8.

[3] Weber F, Knopf H. Incidental findings in magnetic resonance imaging of the brains of healthy young men. J Neurol Sci 2006;240(1-2):81–4.

[4] Wester K. Gender distribution and sidedness of middle fossa arachnoid cysts: a review of cases diagnosed with computed imaging. Neurosurgery 1992;31(5):940–4.

[5] Helland CA, Lund-Johansen M, Wester K. Location, sidedness, and sex distribution of intracranial arachnoid cysts in a population-based sample. J Neurosurg 2010;113 (5):934–9.

[6] Sakai N, et al. Clinical study on intracranial arachnoid cyst: with reference to the middle cranial fossa. No Shinkei Geka 1989;17(2):117–23.

[7] Al-Holou WN, et al. Prevalence and natural history of arachnoid cysts in adults. J Neurosurg 2013;118(2):222–31.

[8] Al-Holou WN, et al. Prevalence and natural history of arachnoid cysts in children Clinical article. J Neurosurg Pediatrics 2010;5(6):578–85.

[9] Rengachary SS, Watanabe I. Ultrastructure and pathogenesis of intracranial arachnoid cysts. J Neuropathol Exp Neurol 1981;40(1):61–83.

[10] Wester K, Pedersen PH. Benign intracerebral cysts treated with internal shunts: review and report of two patients. Neurosurgery 1992;30(3):432–6.

[11] Alaani A, et al. Cerebellopontine angle arachnoid cysts in adult patients: what is the appropriate management? J Laryngol Otol 2005;119(5):337–41.

[12] Boutarbouch M, et al. Management of intracranial arachnoid cysts: institutional experience with initial 32 cases and review of the literature. Clin Neurol Neurosurg 2008;110(1):1–7.

[13] Erman T, et al. Intracranial arachnoid cysts – clinical features and management of 35 cases and review of the literature. Neurosurg Quart 2004;14(2):84–9.

[14] Huang JH, et al. Analysis on clinical characteristics of intracranial Arachnoid Cysts in 488 pediatric cases. Int J Clin Exp Med 2015;8(10):18343–50.

[15] Kandenwein JA, Richter HP, Borm W. Surgical therapy of symptomatic arachnoid cysts – an outcome analysis. Acta Neurochir (Wien) 2004;146(12):1317–22, discussion 1322.

[16] Mottolese C, et al. The parallel use of endoscopic fenestration and a cystoperitoneal shunt with programmable valve to treat arachnoid cysts: experience and hypothesis. J Neurosurg Pediatr 2010;5(4):408–14.

[17] Oertel JM, et al. Endoscopic treatment of arachnoid cysts: a detailed account of surgical techniques and results. Neurosurgery 2010;67(3):824–36.

[18] Park YS, et al. Neurocognitive and psychological profiles in pediatric arachnoid cyst. Childs Nerv Syst 2009;25(9):1071–6.

[19] Spansdahl T, Solheim O. Quality of life in adult patients with primary intracranial arachnoid cysts. Acta Neurochir (Wien) 2007;149(10):1025–32, discussion 1032.

[20] Wang Y, et al. Clinical and radiological outcomes of surgical treatment for symptomatic arachnoid cysts in adults. J Clin Neurosci 2015;22(9):1456–61.

[21] Helland CA, Wester K. Monozygotic twins with mirror image cysts: indication of a genetic mechanism in arachnoid cysts? Neurology 2007;69(1):110−11.

[22] Go KG. The diagnosis and treatment of intracranial arachnoid cysts. Neurosurg Quart 1995;5(3):187−204.

[23] Arriola G, de Castro P, Verdu A. Familial arachnoid cysts. Pediatric Neurol 2005;33 (2):146−8.

[24] Jadeja KJ, Grewal RP. Familial arachnoid cysts associated with oculopharyngeal muscular dystrophy. J Clin Neurosci 2003;10(1):125−7.

[25] Aarhus M, et al. Microarray-based gene expression profiling and DNA copy number variation analysis of temporal fossa arachnoid cysts. Cerebrospinal Fluid Res 2010;7:6.

[26] Helland CA, et al. Increased NKCC1 expression in arachnoid cysts supports secretory basis for cyst formation. Exp Neurol 2010;224(2):424−8.

Molecular Biology and Genetics: Gene Expression, Twin Studies and Familial Occurrence, and Syndromes Associated With AC

Christian A. Helland[1,2]

[1]Haukeland University Hospital, Bergen, Norway
[2]University of Bergen, Bergen, Norway

27

ABBREVIATIONS

ADPKD	autosomal dominant polycystic kidney disease
AM	arachnoid membrane
Aqp	aquaporins
NKCC1	Na-K-Cl cotransporter 1
TSC	tuberous sclerosis complex
qRT-PCR	quantitative real-time polymerase chain reaction

INTRODUCTION

Arachnoid cysts (AC) are regarded as developmental collections of cerebrospinal-like fluid between layers of, or within, the arachnoid. A number of mechanisms have been suggested for their origin and/or their filling: valve mechanisms [1]; meningeal maldevelopment [2–4]; and fluid secretion from the cyst walls [5]. AC exhibit some properties that are not optimally explained on the basis of present theories of cyst development, such as temporal fluctuations of size, growth, and non-trauma related disappearance of the cyst [6–11], see Chapter 10, Classification and Location of Arachnoid Cysts, in this book. The underlying mechanisms of cyst *formation* are however poorly understood and have been so since the first description of this condition by Bright in 1815 [12].

The prevailing theory is that cystogenesis is brought about by a splitting or duplication of the arachnoid membrane during embryogenesis. Cyst fluid may thereafter accumulate either by active water transport across the cyst membrane by the cells lining the cystic cavity, or by a one-way mechanical valve. In both cases, the net flow of water is into the AC. One also has to take into account that there are several features of AC that are not fully covered by these theories alone.

These features include a strong predilection for the middle cranial fossa, a significant male preponderance, and the left-sidedness for cysts in this location [3,11,13,14]. For cysts in the cerebellopontine angle, there is a female preponderance and right-sidedness [15]. These peculiarities and several reports documenting a familial occurrence of AC, either as a separate entity or coexisting with other hereditary disorders [16–27], indicate a genetic mechanism underlying the development of AC as has been suggested by some authors [13,16–18,27,28].

REVIEW OF THE LITERATURE

For this chapter, a search in the PubMed and Web of Science databases was performed. The terms used in the search for the section of genetic mechanisms of cystogenesis and filling were: arachnoid AND cyst AND one of the following terms: "gene*," "gene expression," "genomic," "epigenetic," "gene expression profiling," "reverse transcriptase polymerase chain reaction," "blotting," "microscopy," "(immune) histochemistry," "proteomic," and "transcriptomic." Only original articles written in English, or articles written in other languages with an informative English abstract that described investigation of cyst membrane/fluid in patients with infra- and/or supratentorial intracranial AC in humans were used.

For the section of familial AC and association of AC with hereditary disease/conditions the terms were: arachnoid AND cyst AND one of the following terms: "gene*," "twin*," "monozygotic."

SYNDROMES ASSOCIATED WITH ARACHNOID CYSTS

There are numerous reports of intracranial AC found in patients with different genetic syndromes [16,17,29–41]. However, the cooccurrence of a relatively frequent finding in the general population (AC) [42–44] with a rare syndrome cannot be taken as a proof of causality. On the other side, in some syndromes the prevalence of AC is far higher than in the normal population ($\sim$1%); in these cases it is conceivable that the genetic mechanisms underlying the syndrome might also play a part in the development of AC. An example of this is the coexistence of AC with autosomal dominant polycystic kidney disease (APKD), where cysts in different organs are a hallmark of the condition [20,21,45–48].

For other syndromes, such as tuberous sclerosis complex (TSC), some clinical features (hypomelanotic macules and facial angiofibromas) are likely related to dysfunction of the neural crest. Since the cranial leptomeninges also originate from the neural crest, AC may be expected in TSC. A reported AC prevalence of 5.5% in 220 patients with TSC, along with a male preponderance, supports this assumption [40]. Four patients in this cohort with TSC and AC (33.3%) also had ADPKD due to a contiguous deletion of the TSC2–PKD1 genes [40].

TWIN STUDIES AND FAMILIAL OCCURRENCE

For some locations, AC have been reported to have a familial occurrence, either as an isolated entity, or in covariation with other conditions [16–20,23,25,27,29,37,49–51]. Twin studies are often used to determine the genetic component in various diseases, with the basic assumption that monozygotic twins are genetically identical and hence concordance is indicative of a genetic component.

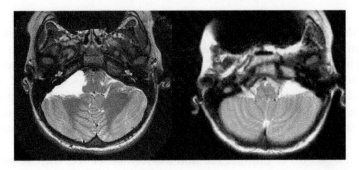

FIGURE 3.1   Axial MR images of symptomatic twin with an arachnoid cyst of the right cerebellopontine angle (left image) and axial MR images of asymptomatic sister with an arachnoid cyst of the left cerebellopontine angle (right image).

Previous twin studies on brain structure have demonstrated a highly heritable component in cerebral and hemispheric volumes [52], but a structural–functional variation in brain structure between monozygotic twins has also been described [53,54]. This variation can also be in the form of mirror imaging [55,56], a chirality that might result from enantiomer information in the very early mammalian embryo [57].

The observation of mirror image cysts in monozygotic twins (Fig 3.1), is thus lending further support to a genetic mechanism in cystogenesis, at least for some AC [58,59].

STUDIES ON GENE EXPRESSION

Given the likely congenital nature of most intracranial AC, it is possible that altered gene expression in neural crest cells at the time of leptomeningeal development may contribute to cyst formation [40].

There has however been a limited amount of research on molecular biology of AC. In their publications, Go et al. demonstrated that the morphological features of the cells lining AC were consistent with fluid secretion capacity [5,60,61]. Moreover, enzyme cytochemistry demonstrated a structural organization of (Na^+-K^+)-ATPase and alkaline phosphatase indicating fluid transport towards the lumen [5].

The later discovery of a family of water-transporting proteins, the aquaporins (Aqp), has given new insight into several physiological and pathological processes concerning water transport in the body, including the brain [62]. In the central nervous system, mainly three Aqps have been identified: Aqp1 in the choroid plexus [63,64]; Aqp4 in the astrocytic end-feet of the blood-brain barrier [62,65,66]; and Aqp9, which was first described in tanycytes and glucose sensitive neurons [67,68]. The role of Aqp has been investigated in cystic diseases in other organs, such as cyst development in ADPKD [69,70]. These findings and publications reporting a higher incidence of AC in patients with ADPKD (8%−10%) [45−47] than in the general population (∼1%) [42,43], made it reasonable to speculate whether Aqps could be involved in the development of AC.

One study trying to link AC and Aqp1 failed to demonstrate Aqp1 immunoreactivity in two AC samples [71]. Moreover, in high-resolution immunogold analysis on AC for the presence of Aqp4 (Fig. 3.2), as part of the investigation of the expression levels of all genes known to be involved in CSF production [72], no evidence for Aqp4 involvement was found, as compared to NKCC1 (Figs. 3.3 and 3.4).

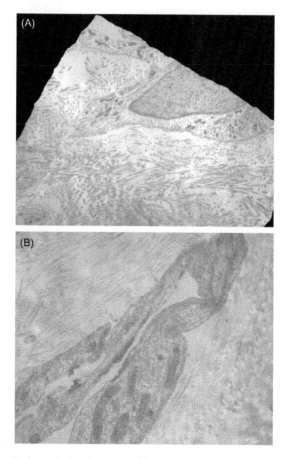

FIGURE 3.2   High-resolution immunogold analysis demonstrates no Aqp4 labeling in the plasma membranes of the cyst-lining cells.

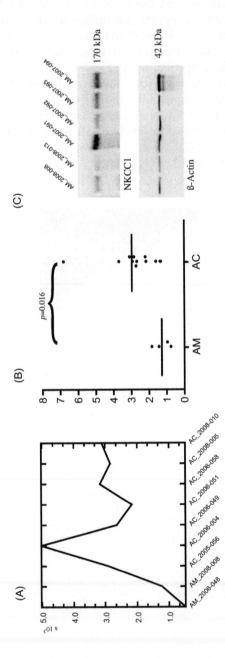

FIGURE 3.3 (A) mRNA expression levels of NKCC1 in AC and normal arachnoid (AM). Gene graph showing the absolute expression values (Y-axis) of the included samples (X-axis) of the NKCC1 gene derived from the mRNA microarray experiment. (B) qRT-PCR of NKCC1 in AC and normal arachnoid (AM) relative to β-actin. The expression was significantly higher in the AC (*P* = .016). (C) Western blots of NKCC1 (170 kDa) in 4 AC samples (AC) and 2 controls (AM) (upper row). Actin (42 kDa) was used as reference protein (lower row). *Reprinted from Helland CA, Aarhus M, Knappskog P, Olsson LK, Lund-Johansen M, Amiry-Moghaddam M, et al. Increased NKCC1 expression in arachnoid cysts supports secretory basis for cyst formation. Exp Neurol. 2010;224(2):424–428 with permission from Elsevier.*

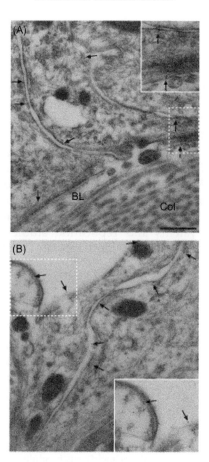

FIGURE 3.4 High-resolution immunogold analysis demonstrate NKCC1 labeling (arrows) appearing as very small dark dots in the plasma membranes of the cyst-lining cells. The labeling is present on the basolateral membranes (A) as well as apical (B) membranes. Higher magnification is shown on the insets. *BL*, basal lamina; *Col*, collagen fibers. Bars: 500 nm. *Reprinted from Helland CA, Aarhus M, Knappskog P, Olsson LK, Lund-Johansen M, Amiry-Moghaddam M, et al. Increased NKCC1 expression in arachnoid cysts supports secretory basis for cyst formation. Exp Neurol. 2010;224(2):424–428 with permission from Elsevier.*

The finding of an upregulation of the CSF-secreting cation chloride cotransporter NKCC1 in AC points to fluid secretion as the main mechanism of AC filling, but does not explain the underlying mechanisms of cystogenesis [72].

The genetic basis in cases with diverse syndromes where the phenotype includes several different features, among them arachnoid cyst, is difficult to elucidate. If the phenotype is unique, a genome-wide linkage study can be performed as a first step. This has been done in a family harboring pachygyria and mental retardation in addition to AC, where a linkage to chromosome 11p15 was demonstrated [41].

In a "pure" arachnoid cyst family, i.e., a family with familial AC occurrence without association to any other syndromes, genome-wide linkage analysis localized the linkage interval to chromosome 6q22.31-23.2 [49]. Other mutations described in connection with AC include *SOX2* mutations [73,74] and *GPSM2* [75], as well as other gene alterations [41,49,73,74,76].

Investigations of gene expression profiles in arachnoid cyst tissue have further identified potential candidate genes underlying cyst formation such as *SHROOM3* and *SOX9* [72,77]. The differential expression of these genes might be important for the development of AC, but due to the low number of cases studied, these findings must be further studied in model systems and replication studies containing more samples before firm conclusions can be made about causality in cyst development.

CONCLUSION

AC demonstrate several features indicating underlying genetic mechanisms for their development, such as familial occurrence and coexistence with other diseases with a known genetic basis for the disease.

References

[1] Dyck P, Gruskin P. Supratentorial arachnoid cysts in adults. A discussion of two cases from a pathophysiologic and surgical perspective. Arch Neurol 1977;34(5):276−9.
[2] Rengachary SS, Watanabe I. Ultrastructure and pathogenesis of intracranial arachnoid cysts. J Neuropathol Exp Neurol 1981;40(1):61−83.
[3] Rengachary SS, Watanabe I, Brackett CE. Pathogenesis of intracranial arachnoid cysts. Surg Neurol 1978;9(2):139−44.
[4] Starkman SP, Brown TC, Linell EA. Cerebral arachnoid cysts. J Neuropathol Exp Neurol 1958;17(3):484−500.
[5] Go KG, Houthoff HJ, Blaauw EH, Havinga P, Hartsuiker J. Arachnoid cysts of the sylvian fissure. Evidence of fluid secretion. J Neurosurg 1984;60(4):803−13.
[6] Becker T, Wagner M, Hofmann E, Warmuth-Metz M, Nadjmi M. Do arachnoid cysts grow? A retrospective CT volumetric study. Neuroradiology 1991;33(4):341−5.
[7] Wester K, Moen G. Documented growth of a temporal arachnoid cyst. J Neurol Neurosurg Psychiatry 2000;69(5):699−700.
[8] Cokluk C, Senel A, Celik F, Ergur H. Spontaneous disappearance of two asymptomatic arachnoid cysts in two different locations. Minim Invasive Neurosurg 2003;46(2):110−12.
[9] Arunkumar MJ, Korah I, Chandy MJ. Dynamic CSF flow study in the pathophysiology of syringomyelia associated with arachnoid cysts of the posterior fossa. Br J Neurosurg 1998;12(1):33−6.

[10] Yamauchi T, Saeki N, Yamaura A. Spontaneous disappearance of temporo-frontal arachnoid cyst in a child. Acta Neurochir (Wien) 1999;141(5):537–40.

[11] Wester K. Peculiarities of intracranial arachnoid cysts: location, sidedness, and sex distribution in 126 consecutive patients. Neurosurgery 1999;45(4):775–9.

[12] Bright R. Serous Cysts in the Arachnoid Diseases of the Brain and Nervous System, Part I: Reports of Medical Cases Selected With a View of Illustrating the Symptoms and Cure of Diseases by a Reference to Morbid Anatomy. London: Longman, Rees, Orme, Brown, and Green; 1831, 1831.

[13] Go KG. The diagnosis and treatment of intracranial arachnoid cysts. Neurosurg Quarterly 1995;5(3):187–204.

[14] Wester K. Gender distribution and sidedness of middle fossa arachnoid cysts – a review of cases diagnosed with computed imaging. Neurosurgery 1992;31(5):940–4.

[15] Helland CA, Lund-Johansen M, Wester K. Location, sidedness, and sex distribution of intracranial arachnoid cysts in a population-based sample. J Neurosurg 2010;113(5): 934–9.

[16] Jadeja KJ, Grewal RP. Familial arachnoid cysts associated with oculopharyngeal muscular dystrophy. J Clin Neurosci 2003;10(1):125–7.

[17] Orlacchio A, Gaudiello F, Totaro A, Floris R, St George-Hyslop PH, Bernardi G, et al. A new SPG4 mutation in a variant form of spastic paraplegia with congenital arachnoid cysts. Neurology 2004;62(10):1875–8.

[18] Arriola G, de Castro P, Verdu A. Familial arachnoid cysts. Pediatr Neurol 2005;33(2): 146–8.

[19] Pomeranz S, Constantini S, Lubetzki-Korn I, Amir N. Familial intracranial arachnoid cysts. Childs Nerv Syst 1991;7(2):100–2.

[20] Alehan FK, Gurakan B, Agildere M. Familial arachnoid cysts in association with autosomal dominant polycystic kidney disease. Pediatrics 2002;110(1 Pt 1):e13.

[21] Leung GK, Fan YW. Chronic subdural haematoma and arachnoid cyst in autosomal dominant polycystic kidney disease (ADPKD). J Clin Neurosci 2005;12(7):817–19.

[22] Tolmie JL, Day R, Fredericks B, Galea P, Moffett AW. Dominantly inherited cerebral dysplasia: arachnoid cyst associated with mild mental handicap in a mother and her son. J Med Genet 1997;34(12):1018–20.

[23] Handa J, Okamoto K, Sato M. Arachnoid cyst of the middle cranial fossa: report of bilateral cysts in siblings. Surg Neurol 1981;16(2):127–30.

[24] Jamjoom ZA, Okamoto E, Jamjoom AH, al-Hajery O, bu-Melha A. Bilateral arachnoid cysts of the sylvian region in female siblings with glutaric aciduria type I. Report of two cases. J Neurosurg 1995;82(6):1078–81.

[25] Sinha S, Brown JI. Familial posterior fossa arachnoid cyst. Childs Nerv Syst 2004;20 (2):100–3.

[26] Wilson WG, Deponte KA, McIlhenny J, Dreifuss FE. Arachnoid cysts in a brother and sister. J Med Genet 1988;25(10):714–15.

[27] Guzel A, Tatli M, Bilguvar K, Diluna ML, Bakkaloglu B, Ozturk AK, et al. Apparently novel genetic syndrome of pachygyria, mental retardation, seizure, and arachnoid cysts. Am J Med Genet A 2007;143(7):672–7.

[28] Hayashi T, Anegawa S, Honda E, Kuramoto S, Mori K, Murata T, et al. Clinical analysis of arachnoid cysts in the middle fossa. Neurochirurgia (Stuttg) 1979;22(6):201–10.

[29] Kurt S, Cevik B, Aksoy D, Sahbaz EI, Gundogdu Eken A, Basak AN. Atypical features in a large turkish family affected with friedreich ataxia. Case Rep Neurol Med 2016;2016:4515938.

[30] Massimi L, Izzo A, Paternoster G, Frassanito P, Di Rocco C. Arachnoid cyst: a further anomaly associated with Kallmann syndrome? Childs Nerv Syst 2016;32(9):1607–14.

[31] Hald JK, Nakstad PH, Skjeldal OH, Stromme P. Bilateral arachnoid cysts of the temporal fossa in four children with glutaric aciduria type I. AJNR Am J Neuroradiol 1991;12(3):407–9.

[32] Yabuki S, Kikuchi S, Ikegawa S. Spinal extradural arachnoid cysts associated with distichiasis and lymphedema. Am J Med Genet A 2007;143A(8):884−7.

[33] Buchino JJ, Nicol KK, Parker Jr. JC. Aicardi syndrome: a morphologic description with particular reference to intracytoplasmic inclusions in cortical astrocytes. Pediatr Pathol Lab Med 1996;16(2):285−91.

[34] Lyons C, Castano G, Jan JE, Sargent M. Optic nerve hypoplasia with intracranial arachnoid cyst. JAAPOS 2004;8(1):61−6.

[35] Yesilkaya E, Karaer K, Bideci A, Camurdan O, Percin EF, Cinaz P. Dubowitz syndrome: a cholesterol metabolism disorder? Genet Couns 2008;19(3):287−90.

[36] Hilal L, Hajaji Y, Vie-Luton MP, Ajaltouni Z, Benazzouz B, Chana M, et al. Unusual phenotypic features in a patient with a novel splice mutation in the GHRHR gene. Mol Med. 2008;14(5-6):286−92.

[37] Odent S, Le Marec B, Toutain A, David A, Vigneron J, Treguier C, et al. Central nervous system malformations and early end-stage renal disease in oro-facio-digital syndrome type I: a review. Am J Med Genet 1998;75(4):389−94.

[38] Holmes LB, Redline RW, Brown DL, Williams AJ, Collins T. Absence/hypoplasia of tibia, polydactyly, retrocerebellar arachnoid cyst, and other anomalies: an autosomal recessive disorder. J Med Genet 1995;32(11):896−900.

[39] Martinez-Lage JF, Poza M, Rodriguez Costa T. Bilateral temporal arachnoid cysts in neurofibromatosis. J Child Neurol 1993;8(4):383−5.

[40] Boronat S, Caruso P, Auladell M, Van Eeghen A, Thiele EA. Arachnoid cysts in tuberous sclerosis complex. Brain Dev 2014;36(9):801−6.

[41] Bilguvar K, Ozturk AK, Bayrakli F, Guzel A, DiLuna ML, Bayri Y, et al. The syndrome of pachygyria, mental retardation, and arachnoid cysts maps to 11p15. Am J Med Genet A 2009;149A(11):2569−72.

[42] Vernooij MW, Ikram MA, Tanghe HL, Vincent AJ, Hofman A, Krestin GP, et al. Incidental findings on brain MRI in the general population. N Engl J Med 2007;357 (18):1821−8.

[43] Weber F, Knopf H. Incidental findings in magnetic resonance imaging of the brains of healthy young men. J Neurol Sci 2006;240(1-2):81−4.

[44] Al-Holou WN, Yew AY, Boomsaad ZE, Garton HJ, Muraszko KM, Maher CO. Prevalence and natural history of arachnoid cysts in children. J Neurosurg Pediatr 2010;5(6):578−85.

[45] Merta M, Rysava R. Brain disorders in autosomal dominant polycystic kidney disease. Sb Lek 1996;97(4):479−85.

[46] Romao EA, Moyses NM, Teixeira SR, Muglia VF, Vieira-Neto OM, Dantas M. Renal and extrarenal manifestations of autosomal dominant polycystic kidney disease. Braz J Med Biol Res 2006;39(4):533−8.

[47] Schievink WI, Huston III J, Torres VE, Marsh WR. Intracranial cysts in autosomal dominant polycystic kidney disease. J Neurosurg 1995;83(6):1004−7.

[48] Wijdicks EF, Torres VE, Schievink WI. Chronic subdural hematoma in autosomal dominant polycystic kidney disease 2. Am J Kidney Dis 2000;35(1):40−3.

[49] Bayrakli F, Okten AI, Kartal U, Menekse G, Guzel A, Oztoprak I, et al. Intracranial arachnoid cyst family with autosomal recessive trait mapped to chromosome 6q22.31-23.2. Acta Neurochir (Wien) 2012;154(7):1287−92.

[50] Hendriks YM, Laan LA, Vielvoye GJ, van Haeringen A. Bilateral sensorineural deafness, partial agenesis of the corpus callosum, and arachnoid cysts in two sisters. Am J Med Genet 1999;86(2):183−6.

[51] Tolmie JL, Day R, Fredericks B, Galea P, Moffett AW. Dominantly inherited cerebral dysplasia: arachnoid cyst associated with mild mental handicap in a mother and her son. J Med Genet 1997;34(12):1018−20.

[52] Bartley AJ, Jones DW, Weinberger DR. Genetic variability of human brain size and cortical gyral patterns. Brain 1997;120(Pt 2):257−69.

[53] Badzakova-Trajkov G, Haberling IS, Corballis MC. Cerebral asymmetries in monozygotic twins: an fMRI study. Neuropsychologia 2010;48(10):3086−93.

[54] Sommer IE, Ramsey NF, Mandl RC, Kahn RS. Language lateralization in monozygotic twin pairs concordant and discordant for handedness. Brain 2002;125(Pt 12): 2710−18.

[55] Sommer IE, Ramsey NF, Bouma A, Kahn RS. Cerebral mirror-imaging in a monozygotic twin. Lancet 1999;354(9188):1445−6.

[56] Gedda L, Brenci G, Franceschetti A, Talone C, Ziparo R. Study of mirror imaging in twins. Prog Clin Biol Res 1981;69A:167−8.

[57] Levin M. Twinning and embryonic left-right asymmetry. Laterality 1999;4(3):197−208.

[58] Helland CA, Wester K. Monozygotic twins with mirror image cysts: indication of a genetic mechanism in arachnoid cysts? Neurology 2007;69(1):110−11.

[59] Zhou JY, Pu JL, Chen S, Hong Y, Ling CH, Zhang JM. Mirror-image arachnoid cysts in a pair of monozygotic twins: a case report and review of the literature. Int J Med Sci 2011;8(5):402−5.

[60] Go KG, Houthoff HJ, Blaauw EH, Stokroos I, Blaauw G. Morphology and origin of arachnoid cysts. Scanning and transmission electron microscopy of three cases. Acta Neuropathol (Berl) 1978;44(1):57−62.

[61] Go KG, Houthoff HJ, Hartsuiker J, Blaauw EH, Havinga P. Fluid secretion in arachnoid cysts as a clue to cerebrospinal fluid absorption at the arachnoid granulation. J Neurosurg 1986;65(5):642−8.

[62] Amiry-Moghaddam M, Ottersen OP. The molecular basis of water transport in the brain. Nat Rev Neurosci 2003;4(12):991−1001.

[63] Longatti P, Basaldella L, Orvieto E, Dei TA, Martinuzzi A. Aquaporin(s) expression in choroid plexus tumours. Pediatr Neurosurg 2006;42(4):228−33.

[64] Longatti PL, Basaldella L, Orvieto E, Fiorindi A, Carteri A. Choroid plexus and aquaporin-1: a novel explanation of cerebrospinal fluid production. Pediatr Neurosurg 2004;40(6):277−83.

[65] Amiry-Moghaddam M, Otsuka T, Hurn PD, Traystman RJ, Haug FM, Froehner SC, et al. An alpha-syntrophin-dependent pool of AQP4 in astroglial end-feet confers bidirectional water flow between blood and brain. Proc Natl Acad Sci USA 2003;100(4): 2106−11.

[66] Amiry-Moghaddam M, Frydenlund DS, Ottersen OP. Anchoring of aquaporin-4 in brain: molecular mechanisms and implications for the physiology and pathophysiology of water transport. Neuroscience 2004;129(4):999−1010.

[67] Agre P, Bonhivers M, Borgnia MJ. The aquaporins, blueprints for cellular plumbing systems. J Biol Chem 1998;273(24):14659−62.

[68] Amiry-Moghaddam M, Lindland H, Zelenin S, Roberg BA, Gundersen BB, Petersen P, et al. Brain mitochondria contain aquaporin water channels: evidence for the expression of a short AQP9 isoform in the inner mitochondrial membrane. FASEB J 2005;19(11):1459−67.

[69] Devuyst O, Beauwens R. Ion transport and cystogenesis: the paradigm of autosomal dominant polycystic kidney disease. Adv Nephrol Necker Hosp 1998;28:439−78.

[70] Longatti P, Basaldella L, Orvieto E, Tos AP, Martinuzzi A. Aquaporin 1 expression in cystic hemangioblastomas. Neurosci Lett 2006;392(3):178−80.

[71] Basaldella L, Orvieto E, Dei Tos AP, Della Barbera M, Valente M, Longatti P. Causes of arachnoid cyst development and expansion. Neurosurg Focus 2007;22(2):E4.

[72] Helland CA, Aarhus M, Knappskog P, Olsson LK, Lund-Johansen M, Amiry-Moghaddam M, et al. Increased NKCC1 expression in arachnoid cysts supports secretory basis for cyst formation. Exp Neurol 2010;224(2):424−8.

[73] Suzuki J, Azuma N, Dateki S, Soneda S, Muroya K, Yamamoto Y, et al. Mutation spectrum and phenotypic variation in nine patients with SOX2 abnormalities. J Hum Genet 2014;59(6):353−6.

[74] Wang P, Liang X, Yi J, Zhang Q. Novel SOX2 mutation associated with ocular coloboma in a Chinese family. Arch Ophthalmol 2008;126(5):709−13.

[75] Doherty D, Chudley AE, Coghlan G, Ishak GE, Innes AM, Lemire EG, et al. GPSM2 mutations cause the brain malformations and hearing loss in Chudley-McCullough syndrome. Am J Hum Genet 2012;90(6):1088−93.

[76] Degerliyurt A, Ceylaner G, Kocak H, Bilginer Gurbuz B, Cihan BS, Rizzu P, et al. A new family with autosomal dominant porencephaly with a novel Col4A1 mutation. Are arachnoid cysts related to Col4A1 mutations? Genet Couns 2012;23(2): 185−93.

[77] Aarhus M, Helland CA, Lund-Johansen M, Wester K, Knappskog PM. Microarray-based gene expression profiling and DNA copy number variation analysis of temporal fossa arachnoid cysts. Cerebrospinal Fluid Res 2010;7:6.

Arachnoid Cysts in Glutaric Aciduria Type I (GA-I)

Nikolas Boy and Stefan Kölker

University Hospital Heidelberg, Heidelberg, Germany

OUTLINE

ABBREVIATIONS

AAM	amino acid mixture
AC	arachnoid cyst
C5DC	glutarylcarnitine
DBS	dried blood spots
GA	glutaric acid
GA-I	glutaric aciduria type I
GCDH	glutaryl-CoA dehydrogenase
GC/MS	gas chromatography/mass spectrometry
MRI	magnetic resonance imaging
MS/MS	tandem mass spectrometry
NBS	newborn screening
3-OH-GA	3-hydroxyglutaric acid
SDH	subdural hemorrhage

Evidence-based recommendations [according to current guideline recommendations [1].

LEVEL OF EVIDENCE I

There is no recommendation at this evidence level for this chapter.

LEVEL OF EVIDENCE II

When GA-I is suspected, diagnostic workup, development of treatment plans, appropriate information, and training of affected individuals and their families should take place in a specialized metabolic center. Affected individuals should be transferred to such centers without delay.

Positive newborn screening results and suggestive clinical, biochemical, and/or neuroradiologic signs should be confirmed by diagnostic workup, including quantitative analysis of GA and 3-OH-GA in urine and/or blood, mutation analysis of GCDH gene, and/or GCDH enzyme analysis in leukocytes or fibroblasts.

Metabolic treatment and regular follow-up monitoring should be implemented by an interdisciplinary team in a specialized metabolic center.

Low lysine diet with additional administration of lysine-free, tryptophan-reduced amino acid mixtures containing essential amino acids is strongly recommended for dietary treatment up to age 6 years.

It is strongly recommended to start emergency treatment without delay and to perform it aggressively during febrile illness, febrile reactions to vaccinations, or perioperative management within the vulnerable period for striatal injury (up to age 6 years).

Neurologic (i.e., epilepsy, movement disorder) or neurosurgical (subdural hemorrhage (SDH)) complications should be managed by a neuropediatrician (later neurologist) and/or neurosurgeon in close cooperation with the metabolic specialist.

INTRODUCTION

Glutaric aciduria type I (GA-I, OMIM #231670), first described in 1975 [2] is an autosomal recessive metabolic disorder of lysine, hydroxlysine, and tryptophan metabolism with an estimated worldwide incidence of 1:110,000 newborns [3,4]. Since the majority of untreated individuals primarily or even exclusively develop neurologic symptoms, GA-I has been termed "cerebral" organic aciduria. Since diagnostic and therapeutic concepts have been optimized during the last decades, neurologic outcome has improved significantly. Evidence-based guidelines for diagnosis and management of GA-I [4a] have recently been revised [1].

GENETICS

GA-I is caused by inherited deficiency of glutaryl-CoA dehydrogenase (GCDH, EC 1.3.8.6). The *GCDH* gene is mapped to chromosome 19p13.2 and encodes a homotetrameric flavin adenine dinucleotide-dependent mitochondrial matrix protein that is involved in degradation of L-lysine, L-hydroxylysine, and L-tryptophan [5,6] catalyzing the dehydrogenation of glutaryl-CoA and the subsequent decarboxylation of enzyme-bound glutaconyl-Co to crotonyl-CoA.

Most patients are compound heterozygous for two different pathogenic *GCDH* gene variations. Five genetic isolates are known with a high carrier frequency (up to 1:10) and incidence (up to 1:250 newborns): the *Old Order Amish Community* in Lancaster County, Pennsylvania, United States [6a], the *Oji-Cree First Nations* in Manitoba and Western Ontario, Canada [7], the *Irish Travellers* in the Republic of Ireland and United Kingdom [8], the *Lumbee* in North Carolina, United States [9], and the *Xhosa* in South Africa [10]. There is evidence for a correlation of the genotype with biochemical parameters and residual enzyme activity but not between the genotype and the clinical phenotype [11–13].

METABOLIC DERANGEMENT

Biochemically, GA-I is characterized by accumulation of glutaric acid (GA), 3-hydroxyglutaric acid (3-OH-GA), glutaconic acid, and glutaryl-carnitine (C5DC) which can be detected in body tissues (blood, urine, and CSF; see *Diagnosis*). Two biochemical subgroups have been arbitrarily delineated based on urinary excretion of GA, i.e., so-called *low* and *high* excretors [14]. Importantly, patients from both biochemical groups show a very similar clinical course during infancy and childhood and, if untreated, both show the same high risk of developing striatal injury [11,13]. However, a recent neuroradiologic study unraveled a higher frequency of white matter abnormalities in high excretors compared to low excretors [15] but clinical relevance on the long-term disease course remains to be determined.

PATHOPHYSIOLOGIC CONCEPTS

The pathomechanism has not yet been fully understood. However, increasing evidence points to an involvement of toxic metabolites disturbing brain energy metabolism and transport of toxic metabolites across biological membranes (Fig. 4.1). Several studies have demonstrated impairment of brain energy metabolism induced by intracerebral accumulation of GA, 3-OH-GA, and glutaryl-CoA: glutaryl-CoA inhibits the 2-oxoglutarate dehydrogenase complex (Krebs cycle enzyme, [17]) and GA impairs the dicarboxylic acid shuttle between astrocytes and neurons [18]. In addition, disturbance of neurotransmission has been demonstrated: 3-OH-GA activates glutamatergic signaling via NMDA receptors [19], and inhibits glutamate uptake from the synaptic clept [20] and glutamate decarboxylase, the key enzyme of GABA synthesis [21].

The blood–brain barrier (BBB) plays a central role in the neuropathogenesis. It was demonstrated in postmortem studies [22,23] and in Gcdh-deficient mice [16,24,25] that GA and 3-OH-GA acids highly accumulate in brain tissue of Gcdh-deficient mice and GA-I patients, noteworthily, to similar extent in both high and low excretors. This is in line with clinical studies highlighting a similar risk of all untreated GA-I patients for manifestation of neurologic disease [13]. The high intracerebral concentrations can be explained by intracerebral de novo synthesis and subsequent accumulation of neurotoxic metabolites due to a limited efflux transport capacity of endothelial organic anion transporter (OAT) at the BBB for dicarboxylic acids such as GA and 3-OH-GA [16,26]. This

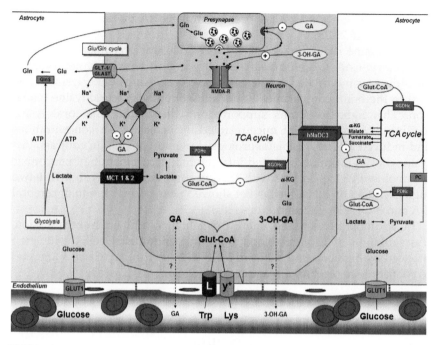

FIGURE 4.1 Synopsis of putative intracerebral pathomechanisms in glutaric aciduria type I. The left-hand side demonstrates the interaction of excitatory (glutamatergic) neurotransmission and cerebral glucose metabolism via the astrocyte–neuron lactate shuttle and the glutamate/glutamine (glu/gln) cycle. The right-hand side presents astrocytic supply of neurons with dicarboxylic TCA cycle intermediates to compensate the continuous drain of a-ketoglutarate required for glutamate synthesis in neurones. The bottom of the illustration presents the BBB (endothelium with tight junctions) and selective transport of hydrophylic nutrients such as L-lysine (Lys) and L-tryptophan (Trp) via specific transporters. L-lysine and L-tryptophan cross the BBB and, subsequently, intracerebral accumulation of glutaryl-CoA, GA, and 3-OH-GA occurs as a result of GCDH deficiency and low permeability of the BBB for dicarboxylic acids (*trapping hypothesis*). Either inhibitory (−) or stimulatory (+) effects of GA, 3-OH-GA, and glutaryl-CoA (Glut-CoA) on different enzymes, receptors, and transporters interfere with the energetic and metabolic coupling between astrocytes and neurones, resulting in an imbalance of glutamatergic neurotransmission and cerebral energy impairment (putative targets for GA, 3-OH-GA, and glutaryl-CoA are shown in red). *GLT-1/GLAST*, sodium dependent astrocytic glutamate transporters; *hNaDC3*, human sodium-dependent dicarboxylate carrier; *Gln*, glutamine; *GlnS*, glutamine synthetase; *Glu*, glutamate; *a-KG*, a-ketoglutaric acid; *KGDHc*, a-ketoglutarate dehydrogenase complex; *MCT 1 and 2*, monocarboxylate transporters 1 and 2; *NMDA-R*, N-methyl-D-aspartate receptor; *Oas*, organic anions; *OAT3*, organic anion transporter; *PC*, pyruvate carboxylase; *PDHc*, pyruvate dehydrogenase complex. *Source: Reprinted from Sauer SW, Okun JG, Fricker G, Mahringer A, Müller I, Crnic LR, et al. Intracerebral accumulation of glutaric and 3-hydroxyglutaric acids secondary to limited flux across the blood–brain barrier constitute a biochemical risk factor for neurodegeneration in glutaryl-CoA dehydrogenase deficiency.* J Neurochem 2006;97:899–910 [16] *with permission from Elsevier.*

pathophysiologic concept has been formulated in the so-called *trapping* hypothesis [16,27,28].

Since lysine is the quantitatively most relevant precursor amino acid for glutaryl-CoA, GA, and 3-OH-GA, it was postulated that neurological outcome was modulated by the amount of oral lysine intake, lysine transport to the brain compartment, and, subsequently, cerebral lysine oxidation. This hypothesis was supported by the finding that oral lysine loading in Gcdh-deficient mice resulted in increased GA concentrations and induced an irreversible neurological phenotype [25]. In contrast, low lysine diet significantly reduced intracerebral accumulation of neurotoxic metabolites [28,29]. In line with this, postmortem investigations in two high excretors on a low lysine diet showed near-normalization of cerebral GA and 3-OH-GA concentrations [30,31].

In addition to impaired energy metabolism and neurotransmission, dysregulation of cerebral blood flow and endothelial cell dysfunction induced by high concentrations of 3-OH-GA in vitro have been suggested to contribute to cerebral disease in GA-I [32,33].

CLINICAL PRESENTATION AND NATURAL DISEASE COURSE

Neonates and infants with GA-I might show nonspecific "soft" neurologic symptoms like muscular hypotonia, feeding difficulties, and delayed motor development, whereas, about half of all patients are asymptomatic. Macrocephaly is frequent (75%) but nonspecific and can be present at or shortly after birth [34,35].

Without treatment, 80%−90% of infants will develop an *acute* encephalopathic crisis during a vulnerable period of brain development (mostly between age 3 and 36 months, with individual reports until age 72 months) which is often precipitated by intercurrent febrile illness, febrile reaction to vaccinations, or surgical intervention [13,36]. The characteristic neurologic sequela of these crises is acute bilateral striatal injury and, subsequently, a complex movement disorder. After the age of 6 years, no crisis has been reported so far.

Using diffusion-weighted MRI, three stages of acute striatal injury have been suggested: (1) an acute stage, within 24 hours of motor regression, characterized by cytotoxic edema within the basal ganglia, cerebral oligemia, and rapid transit of blood throughout the gray matter; (2) a subacute stage, 4−5 days after the onset of clinical signs, characterized by reduced striatal perfusion and glucose uptake, and supervening vasogenic edema; and (3) a chronic stage of striatal atrophy [37]. Within the striatum, neuronal loss spreads in a from ventromedial to dorsolateral direction and mostly affects GABAergic medium-spiny neurons [22], the most abundant neurologic subpopulation of the striatum, resulting in uninhibited tonic inhibition exerted by pallidal neurons and, thus, dystonia.

In addition to the risk for development of movement disorders, risk for epilepsy is also increased in GA-I and even might be the initial presentation [38,39]. As first *extracerebral* manifestations increased frequency of chronic renal failure and peripheral polyneuropathy have been reported in adult patients [40,41].

During the last decades, evidence on variant clinical subtypes, namely *insidious* and *late onset*, has increased, but the use of these terms has been confusing. Patients with *insidious onset* type (10%−20%) develop progressive neurologic symptoms from birth resulting in dystonia and striatal injury in the absence of encephalopathic crises despite early diagnosis and treatment [42,43]. This variant may reflect intrauterine or perinatal neurotoxicity [44,45] and has also been observed in individuals not adhering to current dietary recommendations [45]. *Late onset* GA-I occurs in previously unaffected adolescent/adult patients with nonspecific neurologic symptoms such as headaches, vertigo, transient ataxic gait, polyneuropathy, or reduced fine motor skills but patients do not develop striatal injury. On brain MRI, extrastriatal abnormalities like frontotemporal hypoplasia and periventricular white matter changes are the prominent finding, but also subependymal lesions can occur [45a,46]. Extrastriatal changes are thought to reflect cumulative neurotoxicity [46a]. Also, single cases of neoplastic brain lesions in untreated *late onset* patients [40,47,48] and in one adult patient [49] have been reported. However, whether these findings are coincidental or whether adults with GA-I have an increased risk of (brain) neoplasms—like in L-2-hydroxyglutaric aciduria, another cerebral organic aciduria [50]—is unclear.

Some women with GA-I who have been diagnosed following initially positive newborn screening results of their babies [46a,51,52] have not developed neurological disease despite never having been treated.

DIAGNOSIS

No characteristic or pathognomonic signs or symptoms occurring before acute or insidious onset of complex movement disorder with predominant dystonia are known, making early clinical diagnosis difficult. The characteristic GA-I metabolites GA, 3-OH-GA, glutaconic acid, and glutarylcarnitine (C5DC) can be detected in body fluids (urine, plasma, CSF) and tissues using gas chromatography/mass spectrometry (GC/

MS) or electrospray-ionization tandem mass spectrometry (MS/MS; [14,53]). As neonatal diagnosis and start of treatment significantly improves neurologic outcome in GA-I, the disease has been included in MS/MS-based newborn screening disease panels in many countries [54] but low excretors might be missed due to normal C5DC concentrations [45,55–58]. Pathological NBS results should be confirmed by quantitative analysis of GA and 3-OH-GA in urine and/or blood with GC/MS, mutation analysis of the *GCDH* gene [12,59], and/or GCDH enzyme analysis in leukocytes or fibroblasts [12,14,60]. Diagnosis of GA-I is confirmed by significantly reduced enzyme activity and/or detection of disease-causing mutations on both *GCDH* alleles.

Despite the success of NBS programs as an effective diagnostic intervention, targeted diagnostic workup due to suspicious clinical, laboratory or neuroradiologic signs is still relevant for patients born before the NBS era, in countries without NBS programs or for low excretors that might have been missed by NBS.

NEURORADIOLOGIC ABNORMALITIES

Neuroimaging studies have demonstrated a characteristic pattern of gray and white matter abnormalities in both asymptomatic and symptomatic GA-I patients [37,44,61–66]. Patients after encephalopathic crisis (or patients with *insidious onset* type without an apparent crisis) typically show T2 hyperintensity in putamen, nucleus caudatus, globus pallidus, and ventricles and/or volume loss in the striatum [44,63].

Extrastriatal abnormalities, such as temporal hypoplasia, widening of anterior temporal and sylvian CSF spaces, subependymal pseudocysts, immature gyration pattern, delayed myelination, signal abnormalities in extrastriatal nuclei (thalamus, dentate nuclei, substantia nigra), and isolated T2 hyperintensity in the globus pallidus (Fig. 4.2), frequently occur in all patients *with* and *without* preceding encephalophatic crises, and might regress or even normalize with increasing age if treatment is started in the neonatal period [44].

Some reports on subependymal mass lesions in *late onset* patients have been published [40,46a,47,48], but a causal relationship of the underlying metabolic defect is unclear so far.

Subdural Hemorrhage and Arachnoid Cysts in GA-I

In the infant brain, SDH is caused by tearing of bridging veins in the subdural space due to rotational and decelerating influence. It has been hypothesized for GA-I that microencephalopathic macrocephaly and,

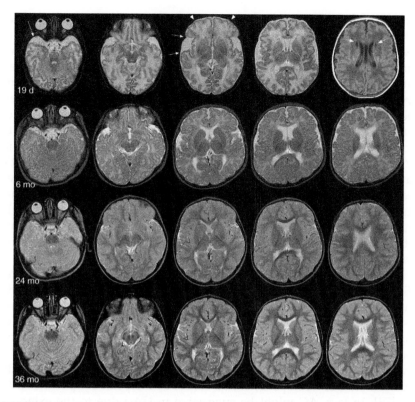

FIGURE 4.2 Sequential MRIs showing extrastriatal abnormalities in a patient with GA-I between the ages of 19 days and 36 months (T2-weighted images, except for fluid attenuated inversion recovery images, right upper corner). MRIs document normalization of frontotemporal hypoplasia (unilateral long arrows) and disappearance of subependymal pseudocysts (short arrows) and cavum vergae. Immature gyration and myelination in the term newborn is characterized by too shallow and less branched sulci (arrowheads) and slightly, diffusely T2 hyperintense white matter. Gyration is adequate for age on follow-up MRIs. Myelination at 24 months is still insufficient in the subcortical temporal and frontal white matter, but at 36 months myelination is complete and the MRI is now normal. *Source: Reprinted from Harting et al. Dynamic changes of striatal and extrastriatal abnormalities in glutaric aciduria type I. Brain 2009;132:1764−1782 [44], with permission from Elsevier.*

subsequently, expanded external CSF spaces increase the risk of stretching bridging veins and thus development of SDH, which may occur after minor accidental head trauma or even spontaneously [66a]. Macrocephaly is present in approximately 70% of both symptomatic and asymptomatic GA-I patients [13]. SDH might appear at any age in GA-I, however, it peaks in late infancy when the extent of macrocephaly is maximal [61,66−71]. It is noteworthy that SDH in GA-I can also occur after minor head trauma even *without* macrocephaly and also in early diagnosed and treated children [72]. This may point to other mechanisms leading to vascular vulnerability and increased risk for SDH. One study demonstrated induction of arteriolar dilation with decreased arterial velocity and elevated cerebral blood volume in GA-I patients, especially between age 13 and 24 months, leading to altered autoregulation, disturbed perfusion pressure and cerebral venous hypertension and subsequently, increased risk for SDH [33]. Moreover, endothelial cell dysfunction induced by intracerebral accumulation of neurotoxic metabolites has been reported which might contribute to increased vascular vulnerability [32]. The exact frequency of SDH in GA-I is unknown since affected individuals may remain asymptomatic but is thought to be rare [73]. SDH in GA-I may be mistaken as abusive head trauma because of chronic or acute subdural and/or retinal hemorrhages [66,68,73,74] and thus, might be a diagnostic pitfall. Importantly, SDH in GA-I is regularly accompanied by additional characteristic neuroradiologic abnormalities of the disease [66]. Therefore, *isolated* SDH per se is not suggestive for GA-I.

Bilateral temporal fluid collections including the anterior temporal CSF spaces and the Sylvian fissure are characteristic for GA-I [75–78]. They may be asymmetric and even space-occupying with hydrocephalus [76]. It has been suggested that these abnormalities might represent bilateral arachnoid cysts [77,78a,78b,78c]. However, this assumption was based on unspecific macroscopic features typical for AC such as a straight medial border of temporal fluid collection [78d]. A recent study reported on four GA-I patients in a cohort of 488 pediatric patients with AC [79]. In fact, AC might be suggestive in GA-I due to the extent of expansive fluid collections and their mass effect on parenchyma. However, it is as yet unknown whether these fluid collections are "true" AC. There is increasing evidence that temporal hypoplasia results from cerebral underdevelopment due to slowed or arrested growth of the temporal lobe during the last trimester of pregnancy [80,81]. Temporal hypoplasia was consistently found in GA-I patients during the newborn period, however, it improved or even completely resolved over time in early diagnosed and treated individuals [44]. Bitemporal AC have been verified in one of two patients on craniotomy [77]. Of note, this patient also suffered from SDH and, therefore, development of a "neomembrane" after SDH mimicking AC might be an alternative explanation. It is also known that GA-I patients who have been diagnosed and treated *late* might develop enlargement and thinning of the skull due to chronic pulsations in CSF spaces (personal communication, I. Harting, Heidelberg) resulting in increased temporal fluid collections. Therefore, it remains to be elucidated whether GA-I patients are really at increased risk for development of bilateral AC.

There have been few reports on GA-I patients who have underwent neurosurgical procedures to treat AC and/or SDH [71,75–78].

Postinterventional outcome was mostly poor, and symptoms were often worsened. However, in many patients with poor outcome the diagnosis GA-I was unclear before neurosurgical intervention and, as a consequence, acute encephalopathic crises were precipitated following inappropriate periinterventional metabolic management. As a consequence, GA-I should be ruled out in pediatric patients with bitemporal AC before any surgical procedure is planned.

TREATMENT AND PROGNOSIS

Today, GA-I is considered to be a treatable condition. Neonatal diagnosis and start of treatment supervised by a specialized metabolic center significantly reduces the frequency of acute encephalopathic crises and movement disorders and increases the probability for an asymptomatic disease course which has been demonstrated by many international studies [3,8,13,37,45,82–88]. Metabolic treatment consists of a low lysine diet with supplementation of a lysine-free, trytophane-reduced, arginine-containing amino acid mixture, oral supplementation of L-carnitine, and an intensified emergency treatment during episodes of intercurrent illness or surgical interventions. It has been recommended by an international guideline group for all patients up to 6 years [4a,89]. Treatment allows normal development and growth [89]. In contrast, therapeutic effectiveness is limited in patients who have been diagnosed after onset of neurologic symptoms [13,34,42,43,90].

The long-term outcome is still incompletely understood; neurologic disease or extracerebral manifestations like chronic kidney disease may occur in adulthood and variable extrastriatal MRI changes may progress after age 6 years [44]. Therefore, protein control using natural protein with a low lysine content and avoidance of lysine-rich food is advisable after age 6 years.

FUTURE PERSPECTIVE

Although details on neuropathology and long-term outcome are still unclear, recent research discoveries as well as a better understanding of phenotype and natural history have led to improved outcomes in GA-I. However, future studies on long-term outcome, treatment monitoring, characterization of variant onset types of GA-I, and methods for reliable detection of low excretors are necessary.

References

[1] Boy N, Mühlhausen C, Maier EM, Heringer J, Assmann B, Burgard P, et al. Proposed recommendations for diagnosing and managing individuals with glutaric aciduria type I: second revision. J Inherit Metab Dis 2017;40:75−101.

[2] Goodman SI, Markey SP, Moe PG, Miles BS, Teng CC. Glutaric aciduria: a 'new' inborn error of amino acid metabolism. Biochem Med 1975;12:12−21.

[3] Kölker S, Garbade SF, Boy N, Maier EM, Meissner T, Mühlhausen C, et al. Decline of acute encephalopathic crises in children with glutaryl-CoA dehydrogenase deficiency identified by neonatal screening in Germany. Pediatr Res 2007;62:353−62.

[4] Lindner M, Kölker S, Schulze A, Christensen E, Greenberg CR, Hoffmann GF. Neonatal screening for glutaryl-CoA dehydrogenase deficiency. J Inherit Metab Dis 2004;27:851−9.

[4a] Kölker S, Christensen E, Leonard JV, et al. Diagnosis and management of glutaric aciduria type I−revised recommendations. J InheritMetab Dis 2011;34:677−94.

[5] Fu Z, Wang M, Paschke R, Rao S, Frerman FE, Kim JJP. Crystal structures of human glutaryl-CoA dehydrogenase with and without an alternate substrate: structural bases of dehydrogenation and decarboxylation reactions. Biochemistry 2004;43: 9674−84.

[6] Greenberg CR, Reimer D, Singal R, Triggs-Raine B, Chudley AE, Dilling LA, et al. A G-to-T transversion at the +5 position of intron 1 in the glutaryl-CoA dehydrogenase gene is associated with the Island Lake variant of glutaric acidemia type I. Hum Mol Genet 1995;4:493−5.

[6a] Morton DH, Bennett MJ, Seargeant LE, Nichter CA, Kelley RI. A common cause of episodic encephalopathy an spastic paralysis in the Amish of Lancaster County, Pennsylvania. Am JMed Genet 1991;41:89−95.

[7] Haworth JC, Booth FA, Chudley AE, deGroot GW, Dilling LA, Goodman SI, et al. Phenotypic variability in glutaric aciduria type I: report of fourteen cases in five Canadian Indian kindreds. J Pediatr 1991;118:52−8.

[8] Naughten ER, Mayne PD, Monavari AA, Goodman SI, Sulaiman G, Croke DT. Glutaric aciduria type I, outcome in the Republic of Ireland. J Inherit Metab Dis 2004;27:917−20.

[9] Basinger AA, Booker JK, Frazier DM, Koeberl DD, Sullivan JA, Muenzer J. Glutaric academia type 1 in patients of Lumbee heritage from North Carolina. Mol Genet Metab 2006;88:90−2.

[10] Van der Watt G, Owen EP, Berman P, Meldau S, Watermeyer N, Olpin SE, et al. Glutaric aciduria type 1 in South Africa-high incidence of glutaryl-CoA dehydrogenase deficiency in black South Africans. Mol Genet Metab 2010;101:178−82.

[11] Christensen E, Ribes A, Merinero B, Zschocke J. Correlation of genotype and phenotype in glutaryl-CoA dehydrogenase deficiency. J Inherit Metab Dis 2004;27:861−8.

[12] Goodman SI, Stein DE, Schlesinger S, Christensen E, Schwartz M, Greenberg CR, et al. Glutaryl-CoA dehydrogenase mutations in glutaric acidemia (Type I): review and report of thirty novel mutations. Hum Mutat 1998;12:141−4.

[13] Kölker S, Garbade S, Greenberg CR, Leonard JV, Saudubray JM, Ribes A, et al. Natural history, outcome, and treatment efficacy in children and adults with glutaryl-CoA dehydrogenase deficiency. Pediatr Res 2006;59:840−7.

[14] Baric I, Wagner L, Feyh P, Liesert M, Buckel W, Hoffmann GF. Sensitivity of free and total glutaric and 3-hydroxyglutaric acid measurement by stable isotope dilution assays for the diagnosis of glutaric aciduria type I. J Inherit Metab Dis 1999;22: 867−82.

[15] Harting I, Boy N, Heringer J, Seitz A, Bendszus M, Pouwels PJ, et al. 1)H-MRS in glutaric aciduria type 1: impact of biochemical phenotype and age on the cerebral accumulation of neurotoxic metabolites. J Inherit Metab Dis 2015;38:829−38.

[16] Sauer SW, Okun JG, Fricker G, Mahringer A, Müller I, Crnic LR, et al. Intracerebral accumulation of glutaric and 3-hydroxyglutaric acids secondary to limited flux across the blood-brain barrier constitute a biochemical risk factor for neurodegeneration in glutaryl-CoA dehydrogenase deficiency. J Neurochem 2006;97:899–910.

[17] Sauer SW, Okun JG, Schwab MA, Crnic LR, Hoffmann GF, Goodman SI, et al. Bioenergetics in glutaryl-coenzyme A dehydrogenase deficiency, a role for glutaryl-coenzyme A. J Biol Chem 2005;280:21830–6.

[18] Lamp J, Keyser B, Koeller DM, Ullrich K, Braulke T, Mühlhausen C. Glutaric aciduria type 1 metabolites impair the succinate transport from astrocytic to neuronal cells. J Biol Chem 2011;286:17777–84.

[19] Kölker S, Köhr G, Ahlemeyer B, Okun JG, Pawlak V, Hörster F, et al. Ca(2+) and Na(+) dependence of 3-hydroxyglutarate-induced excitotoxicity in primary neuronal cultures from chick embryo telencephalons. Pediatr Res 2002;52:199–206.

[20] Porciuncula LO, Dal-Pizzol Jr A, Coitinho AS, Emanuelli T, Souza DO, Wajner M. Inhibition of synaptosomal [³H]glutamate uptake and [³H]glutamate binding to plasma membranes from brain of young rats by glutaric acid in vitro. J Neurol Science 2000;173:93–6.

[21] Stokke O, Goodman SI, Moe PG. Inhibition of brain glutamate decarboxylase by glutarate, gluconate, and beta-hydroxyglutarate: explanation of the symptoms in glutaric aciduria? Clin Chim Acta 1976;66:411–15.

[22] Funk CB, Prasad AN, Frosk P, Sauer S, Kölker S, Greenberg CR, et al. Neuropathological, biochemical, and molecular findings in a glutaric acidemia type 1 cohort. Brain 2005;128:711–22.

[23] Leibel RL, Shih VE, Goodman SI, Bauman ML, McCabe ER, Zwerdling RG, et al. Glutaric acidemia: a metabolic disorder causing progressive choreoathetosis. Neurology 1980;30:1163–8.

[24] Koeller DM, Woontner M, Crnic LS, Kleinschmidt-DeMasters B, Stephens J, Hunt EL, et al. Biochemical, pathological and behavioral analysis of a mouse model of glutaric aciduria type I. Hum Mol Genet 2002;11:347–57.

[25] Zinnanti WJ, Lazovic J, Wolpert EB, Antonetti DA, Smith MB, Connor JR, et al. A diet-induced mouse model for glutaric aciduria type I. Brain 2006;129:899–910.

[26] Hassel B, Brathe A, Petersen D. Cerebral dicarboxylate transport and metabolism studied with isotopically labelled fumarate, malate and malonate. J Neurochem 2002;82:410–19.

[27] Kölker S, Sauer SW, Okun JG, Hoffmann GF, Koeller DM. Lysine intake and neurotoxicity in glutaric aciduria type I: towards a rationale for therapy? Brain 2006;129:e54.

[28] Sauer SW, Opp S, Hoffmann GF, Koeller DM, Okun JG, Kölker S. Therapeutic modulation of cerebral L-lysine metabolism in a mouse model for glutaric aciduria type I. Brain 2011;134:157–70.

[29] Sauer SW, Opp S, Komatsuzaki S, Blank AE, Mittelbronn M, Burgard P, et al. Multifactorial modulation of susceptibility to l-lysine in an animal model of glutaric aciduria type I. Biochim Biophys Acta 2015;1852:768–77.

[30] Bennett MJ, Marlow N, Pollitt RJ, Wales JK. Glutaric aciduria type 1: biochemical investigations and postmortem findings. Eur J Pediatr 1986;145:403–5.

[31] Kölker S, Hoffmann GF, Schor DS, Feyh P, Wagner L, Jeffrey I, et al. Glutaryl-CoA dehydrogenase deficiency: region-specific analysis of organic acids and acylcarnitines in post mortem brain predicts vulnerability of the putamen. Neuropediatrics 2003;34:253–60.

[32] Mühlhausen C, Ott N, Chalajour F, Tilki D, Freudenberg F, Shahhossini M, et al. Endothelial effects of 3-hydroxyglutaric acid: implications for glutaric aciduria type I. Pediatr Res 2006;59:196–202.

[33] Strauss KA, Donnelly P, Wintermark M. Cerebral haemodynamics in patients with glutaryl-coenzyme A dehydrogenase deficiency. Brain 2010;133:76—92.

[34] Bjugstad KB, Goodman SI, Freed CR. Age at symptom onset predicts severity of motor impairment and clinical onset of glutaric aciduria type I. J Pediatr 2000;137:681—6.

[35] Renaud DL. Leukoencephalopathies associated with macrocephaly. Semin Neurol 2012;32:34—41.

[36] Hoffmann GF, Trefz FK, Barth PG, Böhles HJ, Biggemann B, Bremer HJ, et al. Glutaryl-CoA dehydrogenase deficiency: a distinct encephalopathy. Pediatrics 1991;88:1194—203.

[37] Strauss KA, Lazovic J, Wintermark M, Morton DH. Multimodal imaging of striatal degeneration in Amish patients with glutaryl-CoA dehydrogenase deficiency. Brain 2007;130:1905—20.

[38] Kölker S, Cazorla AG, Valayannopoulos V, Lund AM, Burlina AB, Sykut-Cegielska J, et al. The phenotypic spectrum of organic acidurias and urea cycle disorders. Part 1: the initial presentation. J Inherit Metab Dis 2015;38:1041—57.

[39] McClelland VM, Bakalinova DB, Hendriksz C, Singh RP. Glutaric aciduria type1 presenting with epilepsy. Dev Med Child Neurol 2009;51:235—9.

[40] Herskovitz M, Goldsher D, Sela BA, Mandel H. Subependymal mass lesions and peripheral polyneuropathy in adult-onset glutaric aciduria type I. Neurology 2013;81:849—50.

[41] Kölker S, Valayannopoulos V, Burlina AB, Sykut-Cegielska J, Wijburg FA, Teles EL, et al. The phenotypic spectrum of organic acidurias and urea cycle disorders. Part 2: the evolving clinical phenotype. J Inherit Metab Dis 2015;38:1059—74.

[42] Busquets C, Merinero B, Christensen E, Gelpí JL, Campistol J, Pineda M, et al. Glutaryl-CoA dehydrogenase deficiency in Spain: evidence of two groups of patients, genetically and biochemically distinct. Pediatr Res 2000;48:315—22.

[43] Hoffmann GF, Athanassopoulos S, Burlina AB, Duran M, de Klerk JB, Lehnert W, et al. Clinical course, early diagnosis, treatment, and prevention of disease in glutaryl-CoA dehydrogenase deficiency. Neuropediatrics 1996;27:115—23.

[44] Harting I, Neumaier-Probst E, Seitz A, Maier EM, Assmann B, Baric I, et al. Dynamic changes of striatal and extrastriatal abnormalities in glutaric aciduria type I. Brain 2009;132:1764—82.

[45] Heringer J, Boy SPN, Ensenauer R, Assmann B, Zschocke J, Harting I, et al. Use of guidelines improves the neurological outcome in glutaric aciduria type I. Ann Neurol 2010;68:743—52.

[45a] Bähr O, Mader I, Zschocke J, Dichgans J, Schulz J. Adult onset glutaric aciduria type I presenting with a leukoencephalopathy. Neurology 2002;59:1802—4.

[46] Külkens S, Harting I, Sauer S, Zschocke J, Hoffmann GF, Gruber S, et al. Late-onset neurologic disease in glutaryl-CoA dehydrogenase deficiency. Neurology 2005;64: 2142—4.

[46a] Boy N, Heringer J, Brackmann R, Bodamer O, Seitz A, Kölker S, Harting I. Extrastriatal changes in patients with late-onset glutaric aciduria type I Highlight the risk of long-term neurotoxicity. Orphanet J Rare Dis 2017;12:77.

[47] Korman SH, Jakobs C, Darmin PS, Gutman A, van der Knaap MS, Ben-Neriah Z, et al. Glutaric aciduria type 1: clinical, biochemical and molecular findings in patients from Israel. Eur J Paediatr Neurol 2007;11:81—9.

[48] Pierson TM, Nezhad M, Tremblay MA, Lewis R, Wong D, Salamon N, et al. Adult-onset glutaric aciduria type I presenting with white matter abnormalities and subependymal nodules. Neurogenetics 2015;16:325—8.

[49] Burlina AP, Danieli D, Malfa F, Manara R, Del Rizzo M, Bordugo A, et al. Glutaric aciduria type I and glioma: the first report in a young adult patient. J Inherit Metab Dis 2012;35:S1—182.

[50] Patay Z, Mills JC, Löbel U, Lambert A, Sablauer A, Ellison DW. Cerebral neoplasms in L-2 hydroxyglutaric aciduria: 3 new cases and meta-analysis of literature data. AJNR Am J Neuroradiol 2012;33:940−3.

[51] Crombez EA, Cederbaum SD, Spector E, Chan E, Salazar D, Neidich J, et al. Maternal glutaric acidemia type I identified by newborn screening. Mol Genet Metab 2008;94:132−4.

[52] Garcia P, Martins E, Diogo L, Rocha H, Marcão A, Gaspar E, et al. Outcome of three cases of untreated maternal glutaric aciduria type I. Eur J Pediatr 2008;167:569−73.

[53] Chace DH, Kalas TA, Naylor EW. Use of tandem mass spectrometry for multianalyte screening of dried blood specimens from newborns. Clin Chem 2003;40:1797−817.

[54] Loeber JG, Burgard P, Cornel MC, Rigter T, Weinreich SS, Rupp K, et al. Newborn screening programmes in Europe; arguments and efforts regarding harmonization. Part 1. From blood spot to screening result. J Inherit Metab Dis 2012;35:603−11.

[55] Gallagher RC, Cowan TM, Goodman SI, Enns GM. Glutaryl-CoA dehydrogenase deficiency and newborn screening: retrospective analysis of a low excretor provides further evidence that some cases may be missed. Mol Genet Metabol 2005;86:417−20.

[56] Smith WE, Millington DS, Koeberl DD, Lesser PS. Glutaric academia, type I, missed by newborn screening in an infant with dystonia following promethazine administration. Pediatrics 2001;107:1184−7.

[57] Treacy EP, Lee-Chong A, Roche G, Lynch B, Ryan S, Goodman SI. Profound neurological presentation resulting from homozygosity for a mild glutaryl-CoA dehydrogenase mutation with a minimal biochemical phenotype. J Inherit Metab Dis 2003;26:72−4.

[58] Wilcken B, Wiley V, Hammond J, Carpenter Kl. Screening newborns for inborn errors of metabolism by tandem mass spectrometry. N Engl J Med 2003;348:2304−12.

[59] Zschocke J, Quak E, Guldberg P, Hoffmann GF. Mutation analysis in glutaric aciduria type I. J Med Genet 2000;37:177−81.

[60] Christensen E. Improved assay of glutaryl-CoA dehydrogenase in cultured cells and liver: application to glutaric aciduria type I. Clin Chim Acta 1983;129:91−7.

[61] Brismar J, Ozand PT. CT and MR of the brain in glutaric aciemia type I: a review of 59 published cases and a report of 5 new patients. Am J Neuroradiol 1995;16:675−83.

[62] Doraiswamy A, Kesavamurthy B, Ranganatha L. Batwing appearance. A neuroradiologic clue to glutaric aciduria-type 1. Internat J Epil 2015;2:44−8.

[63] Garbade SF, Greenberg CR, Demirkol M, Gökçay G, Ribes A, Campistol J, et al. Unravelling the complex mri pattern in glutaric aciduria type I using statistical models-a cohort study in 180 patients. J Inherit Metab Dis 2014;37:763−73.

[64] Mohammad SA, Abdelkhalek HS, Ahmed KA, Zaki OK. Glutaric aciduria type 1: neuroimaging features with clinical correlation. Pediatr Radiol 2015;45:1696−705.

[65] Singh P, Goraya JS, Ahluwalia A, Saggar K. Teaching NeuroImages: glutaric aciduria type 1 (glutaryl-CoA dehydrogenase deficiency). Neurology 2011;77:e6.

[66] Vester ME, Bilo RA, Karst WA, Daams JG, Duijst WL, van Rijn RR. Subdural hematomas: glutaric aciduria type 1 or abusive head trauma? A systematic review. Forensic Sci Med Pathol 2015;11:405−15.

[66a] Hou LC, Veeravagu A, Hsu AR, et al. Glutaric academia type I: a neurosurgical perspective. J Neurosurg 2007;107:167−72.

[67] Carman KB, Aydogdu SD, Yakut A, Yarar C. Glutaric aciduria type 1 presenting as subdural haematoma. J Paediatr Child Health 2012;48:712.

[68] Hartley LM, Khwaja OS, Verity CM. Glutaric aciduria type 1 and nonaccidental head injury. Pediatrics 2000;107:174−5.

[69] Köhler M, Hoffmann GF. Subdural haematoma in a child with glutaric aciduria type I. Pediatr Radiol 1998;28:582.

[70] Twomey EL, Naughten ER, Donoghue VB, Ryan S. Neuroimaging findings in glutaric aciduria type I. Pediatr Radiol 2003;33:823−30.

[71] Woelfle J, Kreft B, Emons D, Haverkamp F. Subdural hematoma and glutaric aciduria type I. Pediatr Radiol 1996;26:779–81.

[72] Zielonka M, Braun K, Bengel A, Seitz A, Kölker S, Boy N. Severe acute subdural hemorrhage in a patient with glutaric aciduria type I after minor head trauma: a case report. J Child Neurol 2015;30:1065–9.

[73] Vester ME, Visser G, Wijburg F, van Spronsen FJ, Williams M, van Rijn RR. Occurrence of subdural hematomas in Dutch glutaric aciduria type 1 patients. Eur J Pediatr 2016;175:1001–6.

[74] Morris AAM, Hoffmann GF, Naughten ER, Monavari AA, Collins JE, Leonard JV. Glutaric aciduria and suspected child abuse. Arch Dis Child 1999;80:404–5.

[75] Hald JK, Nakstad PH, Skjeldal OH, Stromme P. Bilateral arachnoid cysts of the temporal fossa in four children with glutaric aciduria type I. Am J Neuroradiol 1991;12:407–9.

[76] Jamjoom ZA, Okamoto E, Jamjoom AH, al-Hajery O, Abu-Melha A. Bilateral arachnoid cysts of the sylvian region in female siblings with glutaric aciduria type I. Report of two cases. J Neurosurg 1995;82:1078–81.

[77] Lütcherath V, Waaler PE, Jellum E, Wester K. Children with bilateral temporal arachnoid cysts may have glutaric aciduria type 1 (GAT1); operation without knowing that may be harmful. Acta Neurochir (Wien) 2000;142:1025–30.

[78] Martinez-Lage JF, Casas C, Fernandez MA, Puche A, Rodriguez Costa T, Poza M. Macrocephaly, dystonia, and bilateral temporal arachnoid cysts : glutaric aciduria type 1. Childs Nerv Syst 1994;10:198–203.

[78a] Jamjoom ZA, Okamoto E, Jamjoom AH, Al-Hajery O, Abu-Melha A. Bilateral arachnoid cysts of the sylvian region in female siblings with glutaric aciduria type I. Report of two cases. J Neurosurg 1995;82:1078–81.

[78b] Martinez-Lage JF, Casas C, Fernandez MA, Puche A, Costa T Rodriguez, Poza M. Macrocephaly, dystonia, and bilateral temporal arachnoid cysts: glutaric aciduria type 1. Childs Nerv Syst 1994;10:198–203.

[78c] Renner C, Razeghi S, Uberall MA, Hartmann P, Lehnert W. Clinically asymptomatic glutaric aciduria type I in a 4 5/12-year-old girl with bilateral temporal arachnoid cysts. J Inherit Metab Dis 1997;20:840–1.

[78d] Banna M. Arachnoid cysts on computed tomography. AJR Am J Roentgenol 1976;127:979–82.

[79] Huang JH, Mei WZ, Chen Y, Chen JW, Lin ZX. Analysis on clinical characteristics of intracranial Arachnoid Cysts in 488 pediatric cases. Int J Clin Exp Med 2015;8: 18343–50.

[80] Lin SK, Hsu SG, Ho ES, Tsai CR, Hseih YT, Lo FC, et al. Novel mutations and prenatal sonographic findings of glutaric aciduria (type I) in two Taiwanese families. Prenat Diagn 2002;22:725–9.

[81] Mellerio C, Marignier S, Roth P, Gaucherand P, des Portes V, Pracros JP, et al. Prenatal cerebral ultrasound and MRI findings in glutaric aciduria Type 1: a de novo case. Ultrasound Obstet Gynecol 2008;31:712–14.

[82] Couce ML, López-Suárez O, Bóveda MD, Castiñeiras DE, Cocho JA, García-Villoria J, et al. A Glutaric aciduria type I: outcome of patients with early- versus late-diagnosis. Eur J Paediatr Neurol 2013;17:383–9.

[83] Bijarnia S, Wiley V, Carpenter K, Christodoulou J, Ellaway CJ, Wilcken B. Glutaric aciduria type I: out come following detection by newborn screening. J Inherit Metab Dis 2008;31:503–7.

[84] Lee CS, Chien YH, Peng SF, Cheng PW, Chang LM, Huang AC, et al. Promising outcomes in glutaric aciduria type I patients detected by newborn screening. Metab Brain Dis 2013;28:61–7.

[85] Boneh A, Beauchamp M, Humphrey M, Watkins J, Peters H, Yaplito-Lee J. Newborn screening for glutaric aciduria type I in Victoria: treatment and outcome. Mol Genet Metab 2008;94:287−91.

[86] Strauss KA, Puffenberger EG, Robinson DL, Morton DH. Type I glutaric aciduria, part 1: natural history of 77 patients. Am J Med Genet 2003;121C:38−52.

[87] Strauss KA, Brumbaugh J, Duffy A, Wardley B, Robinson D, Hendrickson C, et al. Safety, efficacy and physiological actions of a lysine-free, arginine-rich formula to treat glutaryl-CoA dehydrogenase deficiency: focus on cerebral amino acid influx. Mol Genet Metab 2011;104:93−106.

[88] Viau K, Ernst SL, Vanzo RJ, Botto LD, Pasquali M, Longo N. Glutaric acidemia type 1: outcomes before and after expanded newborn screening. Mol Genet Metab 2012;106: 430−8.

[89] Boy N, Haege G, Heringer J, Assmann B, Mühlhausen C, Ensenauer R, et al. Low lysine diet in glutaric aciduria type I-effect on anthropometric and biochemical follow-up parameters. J Inherit Metab Dis 2013;36:525−33.

[90] Kyllerman M, Skjeldal O, Christensen E, Hagberg G, Holme E, Lönnquist T, et al. Long-term follow-up, neurological outcome and survival rate in 28 Nordic patients with glutaric aciduria type 1. Eur J Paediatr Neurol 2004;8:121−9.

5

Ultrastructure of Arachnoid Cysts

Katrin Rabiei[1,2] and Bengt R. Johansson[2]

[1]Sahlgrenska University Hospital, Gothenburg, Sweden [2]University of Gothenburg, Gothenburg, Sweden

ABBREVIATIONS

AQP-1 aquaporin-1
CEA carcinoembryonic antigen

Arachnoid Cysts: Epidemiology, Biology, and Neuroimaging
DOI: http://dx.doi.org/10.1016/B978-0-12-809932-2.00005-3

CNS	central nervous system
CSF	cerebrospinal fluid
EMA	epithelial membrane antigen
EM	electron microscopy
LM	light microscopy
GFAP	glial fibrillary acidic protein
VIM	vimentin

INTRODUCTION

The morphology of tissues relates to their functional properties. While light microscopic (LM) examination of tissues is the most used method in clinical practice, electron microscopic (EM) examinations provide much more complex and detailed information on intra- and extra-cellular organization of the specimen. Arachnoid cyst (AC) wall morphology was first described with LM in the 1960s [1,2]. In the first reports of their ultrastructure the AC wall was found to be similar to that of the normal arachnoid membrane with a few exceptions [3,4]. However, later reports show that not all cysts classified as ACs have the arachnoid-like morphology [5,6].

This chapter is a brief account on the present knowledge of AC ultrastructure, including comments on other cystic malformations encountered in the subarachnoid space.

ULTRASTRUCTURE OF THE ARACHNOID MEMBRANE

In adults, the arachnoid membrane consists of three layers. The first one, the outer mesothelial layer, consists of up to six layers of closely packed flattened meningeal cells with a barrier function [7]. This layer is lined by a more or less continuous basement membrane, and the cells here are connected by desmosomes. The thickness of the outer cell layer varies greatly in different regions of the CNS. In areas where this layer is particularly thick, so-called "meningothelial nests," cytoplasmic whorls and psammoma bodies are found. Arachnoid cells of this layer have a myriad of branching cytoplasmic processes, which form concentric whorls. The processes are separated by intercellular spaces and connected by gap junctions and desmosomes.

The second layer consists of trabecular connective tissue. This layer also varies in thickness and fiber density in different areas. There are usually very few cells in this layer and fibroblasts are absent. Traversing trabeculae arise from this layer and attach the arachnoid to the pia.

The inner subdivision of the arachnoid, the reticular layer, consists of more loosely arranged, and less flattened cells [8,9]. These cells are linked by gap junctions and desmosomes, which also link the cells of this layer to the cells of the outer layer of the arachnoid membrane. The innermost CSF-facing cells have a more flattened and elongated appearance forming an epithelial-like lining [10,11].

Examined with scanning electron microscopy (SEM), the subdural arachnoid cell layer is arranged like cobblestones, while the inner cell layer has a cobweb appearance because of the cell processes.

IMMUNOHISTOCHEMISTRY OF AC

Immunohistochemical staining of AC wall is described in a few cases. Studying five cases of AC stained for epithelial membrane antigen (EMA), glial fibrillary acidic protein (GFAP), carcinoembryonic antigen (CEA), S-100, and prealbumin, Inoue et al. found ACs to only be positive for EMA [12]. Another study found in addition that ACs were also positive for Vimentin (VIM) [13]. However, the presence of Aquaporin-1 (AQP-1) has not been demonstrated in ACs [14]. However, cysts located in subarachnoid space have also been shown to express both cytokeratin and CEA [15,16].

Expression of hormonal receptors has also been studied in ACs. Immunohistochemical staining has demonstrated the presence of progesterone receptors in the AC wall. However, unlike meningioma cells, the presence of estrogen- or androgen receptors has not been shown in ACs [17,18].

ULTRASTRUCTURE OF AC

AC ultrastructure has originally been described to be similar to that of the normal arachnoid membrane with a few differences. The collagenous reinforcement of the connective tissue layer of the AC wall and the absence of traversing trabeculae were described as the main differences between the structures of the cyst membrane compared to the normal arachnoid [9]. However, there have been many case reports of ACs or cysts located in the subarachnoid space with a different morphology than the classic description of the ACs [19,20]. These cysts have been shown to display features and share many similarities with other intracranial cysts such as colloid cysts, epithelial cysts and glioependymal cysts [15,16,21]. The compelling evidence to this day suggests that in fact some of the cysts classically labeled as ACs based on their

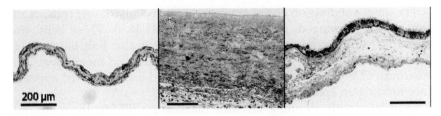

FIGURE 5.1 Light microscopic view of the different types of cyst wall with Richardson's stain. All scale bars are 200 μm. Left: type I, "arachnoid-like type." Middle: type II, "connective tissue type." Right: type III, "aberrant type" of AC.

radiological appearance and subarachnoid localization, may share more similarities with these other cystic malformations in the central nervous system than with the classical ACs [5].

In a prospective setting we attempted to systematically study the detailed EM morphology of cysts located in subarachnoid space and with a radiological and histopathological diagnosis of AC. The findings of the study confirm the diverse nature of cystic malformations in the subarachnoid space. We arrived at the tentative conclusion that at least three types of morphological appearance can be found in cystic lesions of the brain. It should be emphasized that even with LM examinations the differences between the cysts are apparent considering the thickness of the cyst wall, cellularity, and vascularization (Fig. 5.1) [5].

The ultrastructural characterization of these three cyst types is summarized in Table 5.1 and in the text below.

ACs WITH ARACHNOID-LIKE MORPHOLOGY (TYPE I)

ACs of this group compare to normal arachnoid tissue with a few exceptions as described by Rengachary and Watanabe [9]. In these cysts a multilayered subdural meningothelium forms complex cellular extensions in whorls with wide extracellular spaces (Fig. 5.2 upper row). Examination with SEM reveals a smooth continuous surface. The core of the cyst wall consists of a trabecular connective tissue with widely spaced cells and scattered microvessels. A single layer of flattened epithelial cells with organized junctions and a moderate number of short microvilli line the luminal side of the cyst. Regions of multilayered arachnoid epithelium occur just as they do in normal arachnoid tissue. A duplication of the arachnoid membrane is the most probable explanation for this type of cyst.

TABLE 5.1   Morphological Characteristics of the Cysts of the Different Groups

Morphological Characteristic	Type I	Type II	Type III
Thickness	20–150 μm	30–800 μm	6–400 μm
Connective tissue	Thin	Thick layer that constitutes major part of the cyst wall	Thin
Meningothelial epithelium	Present on both sides	Sparsely present	Present in some on dural side
Luminal surface	One to multiple layers	Single layer	Stratified or single layer
Presence of ciliated cells	Not present	Not present	Often present
Presence of microvilli	Sparse	Sparse	Abundant
Glial cell processes	Not present	Not present	Often present

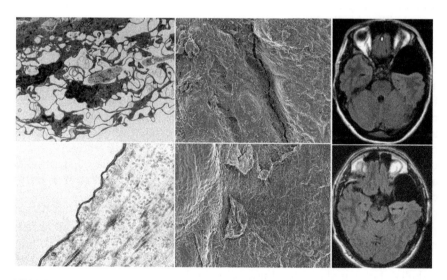

FIGURE 5.2   Upper row: type I ("arachnoid-like") AC. Left: TEM image with a typical meningothelial epithelium on the outer layer of the arachnoid membrane. Middle: SEM image of the outer layer of the same cyst. Right: MRI of the corresponding cyst. Lower row: type II ("connective tissue type") AC. Left: TEM image of the luminal side of an AC. Middle: SEM image of the same cyst. Right: MRI of the corresponding cyst.

ARACHNOID CYSTS WITH FIBROUS MORPHOLOGY (TYPE II)

ACs in this group are generally similar to the cysts in with an arachnoid-like morphology with one important exception. These cysts are generally thicker with a dominating core of dense connective tissue and scarce cellular elements. The epithelium on both aspects of the cyst is single-layered with preserved meningothelial appearance on the subdural side. The luminal aspect could indicate some desquamation of cells and shows few microvilli (Fig. 5.2 lower row).

ARACHNOID CYSTS WITH ABERRANT MORPHOLOGY (TYPE III)

This heterogeneous category can perhaps be subdivided further into groups because of the unique characteristics some of the cysts in this group display. Common properties shared among these cysts were a luminal surface richly equipped with microvilli of uniform length. In four of the eight cysts in this group the luminal epithelium also contained ciliated cells. These cysts shared common characteristics with colloid cysts, glioependymal cysts and epithelial cysts [15,20–23]. The ciliated cells can cover the luminal side of the cyst wall either as sharply delineated patches in varying degrees or completely. Ciliated cells can also be isolated in an environment of microvilli-rich cells (Fig. 5.3). From their apical surface the ciliated cells can also project long slender microvilli, which lack the surface coating of the uniform blunt microvilli in neighboring cells. The apical cytoplasm of ciliated cells can be rich in mitochondria or exhibit apical accumulations of possible secretory granules with electron-dense content (Fig. 5.4). As a rule, the ciliated cells are incorporated into an epithelium with several cell layers and well-developed intercellular junctional complexes. Cysts can also have a complex packing of unmyelinated nerve fibers in their subepithelial position or networks of cellular processes with highly condensed masses of cytoskeletal fibrils indicating a glial nature forming a substantial part of the cyst wall (Fig. 5.4). These latter cells are mostly subepithelial, but can also extend into a lumen-lining position.

DIFFERENTIAL DIAGNOSIS

Ependymal cysts, choroid plexus cysts, and neuroependymal or glioependymal cysts are all intracranial cysts, constituting differential

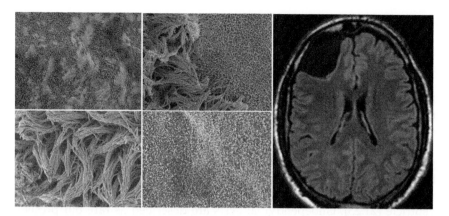

FIGURE 5.3 SEM image of the luminal side of the aberrant type of arachnoid cyst (type III). Upper left: The epithelium exhibits a mosaic of two cell types, one with numerous cilia, and another with a myriad of microvilli. Upper middle: Detailed image of the specimen (5000X magnification). Lower left: Luminal surface cilia. Lower middle: Microvilli. Far right: MRI of the corresponding cyst.

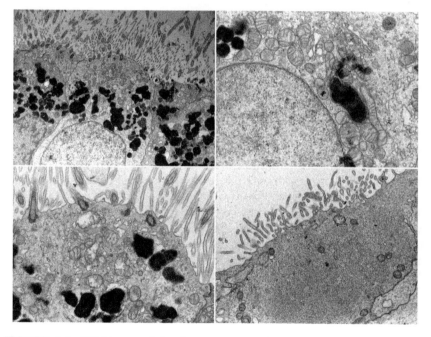

FIGURE 5.4 TEM images of the aberrant cyst type. Upper row (left and middle) and lower row left: Microvilli and cilia of the luminal side of the cyst. Numerous irregular vesicles with electron-dense content are seen in the cytoplasm. The cytoplasm is rich in mitochondria. Lower row, right: Another cyst where the cytoplasm is almost completely occupied with masses of intermediate filaments. In this image, a filament-rich cell with brush border-like microvilli towards the cyst lumen is seen.

diagnoses of AC. Ependymal cysts have been described as being located deep in the brain parenchyma and lined with cuboidal epithelium [24]. Most ependymal cysts are asymptomatic and only very few become symptomatic [25].

Choroid plexus cysts are located in the ventricles or originate from the ventricle and extend into the parenchyma. They contain tissue from the choroid plexus and are mostly located bilaterally. Symptomatic choroid plexus cysts are rare [25].

Glioependymal cysts are also called neuroectodermal cysts or neuroglial cysts and are lined with epithelial lining or endodermal-like epithelial lining [20,22,24,26]. Many of the cysts described in the literature share some morphological characteristics with colloid cysts of the third ventricle [21,23]. Glioependymal cysts are described as rare but present along the entire neuroaxis. These cysts are mostly located within the brain parenchyma, but have also been described in the subarachnoid space [20,25,27]. Friede and Yasargil postulated that these cysts originated from the wall of the neural tube [23].

SUMMARY

ACs were originally described to share more similarities with arachnoid membrane than they do exhibit differences. However, later morphological and/or immunohistochemical analyses of the AC wall revealed that several different types of cyst reside in the subarachnoid space [28,29]. Based on a systematic study of the ACs and on the available literature, we argue that ACs are not a single entity. The morphological appearance of ACs shows that some cysts share common characteristics with glioependymal and colloid cysts [5,15,16,29]. This might in fact have a bearing on expansion mechanisms as well as the clinical behavior of these cysts. While many ACs are indolent, some, which are labeled as ACs due to their location and radiological appearance, share morphological characteristics, and perhaps possess expansion mechanisms of other types of cysts in the central nervous system. With the further development of radiological methods in the future, the aberrant cysts might be distinguished and separated from "true" ACs, i.e., originating from the arachnoid anlage.

References

[1] Lewis AJ. Infantile hydrocephalus caused by arachnoid cyst. Case report. J Neurosurg 1962;19:431–4. Available from: http://dx.doi.org/10.3171/jns.1962.19.5.0431.

[2] Gardner WJ, Mc CL, Dohn DF. Embryonal atresia of the fourth ventricle. The cause of "arachnoid cyst" of the cerebellopontine angle. J Neurosurg 1960;17:226−37. Available from: http://dx.doi.org/10.3171/jns.1960.17.2.0226.

[3] Rengachary SS, Watanabe I, Brackett CE. Pathogenesis of intracranial arachnoid cysts. Surg Neurol 1978;9(2):139−44.

[4] Go KG, Houthoff HJ, Blaauw EH, Stokroos I, Blaauw G. Morphology and origin of arachnoid cysts. Scanning and transmission electron microscopy of three cases. Acta Neuropathol 1978;44(1):57−62.

[5] Rabiei K, Tisell M, Wikkelso C, Johansson BR. Diverse arachnoid cyst morphology indicates different pathophysiological origins. Fluids Barriers CNS 2014;11(1):5. Available from: http://dx.doi.org/10.1186/2045-8118-11-5.

[6] Schuhmann MU, Tatagiba M, Hader C, Brandis A, Samii M. Ectopic choroid plexus within a juvenile arachnoid cyst of the cerebellopontine angle: cause of cyst formation or reason of cyst growth. Pediatr Neurosurg 2000;32(2):73−6 http://dx.doi.org/28902.

[7] Haines DE, Harkey HL, Al-Mefty O. The "subdural" space: a new look at an outdated concept. Neurosurgery 1993;32(1):111−20.

[8] Nabeshima S, Reese TS, Landis DM, Brightman MW. Junctions in the meninges and marginal glia. J Comp Neurol 1975;164(2):127−69. Available from: http://dx.doi.org/10.1002/cne.901640202.

[9] Rengachary SS, Watanabe I. Ultrastructure and pathogenesis of intracranial arachnoid cysts. J Neuropathol Exp Neurol 1981;40(1):61−83.

[10] Adeeb N, Deep A, Griessenauer CJ, Mortazavi MM, Watanabe K, Loukas M, et al. The intracranial arachnoid mater: a comprehensive review of its history, anatomy, imaging, and pathology. Childs Nerv Syst 2013;29(1):17−33. Available from: http://dx.doi.org/10.1007/s00381-012-1910-x.

[11] Vandenabeele F, Creemers J, Lambrichts I. Ultrastructure of the human spinal arachnoid mater and dura mater. J Anat 1996;189(Pt 2):417−30.

[12] Inoue T, Matsushima T, Fukui M, Iwaki T, Takeshita I, Kuromatsu C. Immunohistochemical study of intracranial cysts. Neurosurgery 1988;23(5):576−81.

[13] Morimura T, Maeda Y, Tani E, Nishigami T. Immunohistochemical differential diagnosis of benign cysts in the central nervous system. Noshuyo Byori 1994;11(1):7−13.

[14] Basaldella L, Orvieto E, Dei Tos AP, Della Barbera M, Valente M, Longatti P. Causes of arachnoid cyst development and expansion. Neurosurg Focus 2007;22(2):E4.

[15] Ho KL, Chason JL. Subarachnoid epithelial cyst of the cerebellum. Immunohistochemical and ultrastructural studies. Acta Neuropathol 1989;78(2):220−4.

[16] Akaishi K, Hongo K, Ito M, Tanaka Y, Tada T, Kobayashi S. Endodermal cyst in the cerebellopontine angle with immunohistochemical reactivity for CA19-9. Clin Neuropathol 2000;19(6):296−9.

[17] Leaes CG, Meurer RT, Coutinho LB, Ferreira NP, Pereira-Lima JF, da Costa Oliveira M. Immunohistochemical expression of aromatase and estrogen, androgen and progesterone receptors in normal and neoplastic human meningeal cells. Neuropathology 2010;30(1):44−9. Available from: http://dx.doi.org/10.1111/j.1440-1789.2009.01047.x.

[18] Go KG, Blankenstein MA, Vroom TM, Blaauw EH, Dijk F, Hollema H, et al. Progesterone receptors in arachnoid cysts. An immunocytochemical study in 2 cases. Acta Neurochir (Wien) 1997;139(4):349−54.

[19] Miyagami M, Kasahara E, Miyazaki S, Tsubokawa T, Kagawa Y. Ultrastructural findings of arachnoid cysts and epithelial cysts. No To Shinkei 1991;43(6):545−53.

[20] Tandon PN, Roy S, Elvidge A. Subarachnoid ependymal cyst. Report of two cases. J Neurosurg 1972;37(6):741−5.

[21] Ghatak NR, Kasoff I, Alexander E. Further observation on the fine structure of a colloid cyst of the third ventricle. Acta Neuropathol 1977;39(2):101−7.

[22] Hirai O, Kondo A, Kusaka H. Endodermal epithelial cyst in the prepontine cistern extending into the fourth ventricle—case report. Neurol Med Chir (Tokyo) 1991;31 (5):283−6.

[23] Friede RL, Yasargil MG. Supratentorial intracerebral epithelial (ependymal) cysts: review, case reports, and fine structure. J Neurol Neurosurg Psychiatry 1977;40 (2):127−37.

[24] Hirano A, Hirano M. Benign cystic lesions in the central nervous system. Light and electron microscopic observations of cyst walls. Childs Nerv Syst 1988;4(6):325−33.

[25] Osborn AG, Preece MT. Intracranial cysts: radiologic-pathologic correlation and imaging approach. Radiology 2006;239(3):650−64. Available from: http://dx.doi.org/10.1148/radiol.2393050823.

[26] Hirai O, Kawamura J, Fukumitsu T. Prepontine epithelium-lined cyst. Case report. J Neurosurg 1981;55(2):312−17. Available from: http://dx.doi.org/10.3171/jns.1981.55.2.0312.

[27] Lara M, Pascual D, Aparicio MA, Ruiz L, Miranda D, Gomez-Moreta JA, et al. Giant and recurrent enterogenous cyst of the frontal lobe: case report. Childs Nerv Syst 2011;27(8):1333−9. Available from: http://dx.doi.org/10.1007/s00381-011-1463-4.

[28] Leung SY, Ng TH, Fung CF, Fan YW. An epithelial cyst in the cerebellopontine angle. Case report. J Neurosurg 1991;74(2):278−82. Available from: http://dx.doi.org/10.3171/jns.1991.74.2.0278.

[29] Christov C, Chretien F, Brugieres P, Djindjian M. Giant supratentorial enterogenous cyst: report of a case, literature review, and discussion of pathogenesis. Neurosurgery 2004;54(3):759−63 discussion 763.

Pathophysiology of Intracranial Arachnoid Cysts: Hypoperfusion of Adjacent Cortex

Spyridon Sgouros[1,2] and Christos Chamilos[1]

[1]"Mitera" Childrens Hospital, Athens, Greece
[2]University of Athens, Athens, Greece

ABBREVIATIONS

AC arachnoid cyst
CSF cerebrospinal fluid
CT computerized tomography
ICP intracranial pressure
MR magnetic resonance

Arachnoid Cysts: Epidemiology, Biology, and Neuroimaging
DOI: http://dx.doi.org/10.1016/B978-0-12-809932-2.00006-5

INTRODUCTION

Arachnoid cysts (ACs) of the central nervous system are a relatively common neurodevelopmental disorder with an estimated prevalence of 0.2%–2.6% [1–3]. A recent large study of 11,738 brain magnetic resonance (MR) scans of patients aged 18 years and under revealed the presence of an AC in 309 individuals, a prevalence of 2.6%, with a strong male preponderance [1]. ACs appear more frequently in the middle cranial fossa, but can be found in many other locations of the brain and spine as well, and preliminary data indicate genetic mechanisms are involved in their formation [4]. Most cysts appear to be expansive, as they cause a midline shift or compression of nearby cerebral tissue or cerebrospinal fluid (CSF) compartments. ACs are nowadays detected more often, as neuroimaging is used more frequently. Many times they are discovered as incidental findings at scans performed for other reasons [1]. Patients with intracranial ACs may have only mild symptoms from the cyst, even if the cyst is large, and cognition and neurological functions appear normal. This reflects the brain's ability to compensate for slow changes of volume and pressure. When clinical symptoms are present, the most frequent are symptoms of raised intracranial pressure, such as headache and dizziness [5]. Rarely, an AC can cause cranial nerve compression, such as sixth and twelfth nerve compression (from a cyst in the posterior fossa) [6,7]. All these symptoms are reversible after surgical decompression of the cyst. Convulsive episodes have been reported in association with ACs but it remains controversial if these are directly due to the cysts, and some surgeons do not regard epilepsy as an indication for surgical treatment, and often epilepsy does not improve after successful surgical decompression of the cyst, see also Chapter 3, Intracranial Arachnoid Cysts and Epilepsy, of Volume 2.

Overall improvements of quality of life, as well as cognitive functions, have been observed in most patients following successful treatment of intracranial ACs [8–10], see Chapter 16, Pre- and Postoperative Quality of Life in Arachnoid Cyst Patients, of Volume 2. It is interesting that in the large study of incidentally discovered cerebral ACs, in up to 80% of patients the ACs do not enlarge with time and patients who were discovered over the age of 4 years did not develop any subsequent enlargement of the cyst [1], see Chapter 11, Growth and Disappearance of Arachnoid Cysts.

INFLUENCE OF ARACHNOID CYST ON BRAIN FUNCTION

Intracranial Hypertension

Elevated Intracranial Pressure (ICP) caused by the increased volume of the cyst can compromise the function of the adjacent cerebral cortex. Studies in pediatric patients found an increased ICP only in patients with large cysts, and a normal ICP in children with smaller type I cysts [11,12]. Correlation between intracystic pressure and preoperative symptoms has been demonstrated in some studies [13]. Other studies in the adult population have not demonstrated a clear correlation between ICP and symptoms. Certainly, large middle fossa ACs can cause a shift of midline structures and signal change in the underlying white matter of the hemisphere, all indications of raised ICP (Figs. 6.1 and 6.2).

It is uncertain if the intracranial hypertension caused by ACs influences the compliance of the brain, which could lead to pathological CSF pressure wave amplitudes and reduced vascular pulsatility.

Several reports exist of patients with psychiatric manifestations, who were found to have ACs and who settled symptomatically after successful surgical treatment of the AC [14,15], see Chapter 6, Intracranial Arachnoid Cysts And Mental Functions, of Volume 2. Whilst this is unusual, it raises the question as to what extent the presence of the cyst influences global brain function, beyond the obvious connection with intracranial hypertension, as psychiatric symptoms are not a manifestation of raised ICP traditionally.

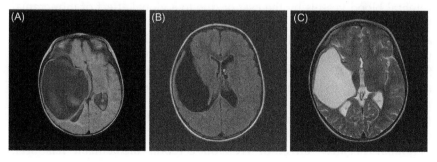

FIGURE 6.1   MR images of an 8-month-old child with increasing head circumference and vomiting and a large right middle fossa AC. (A) Flair axial, at presentation. (B) Flair axial after successful endoscopic fenestration. (C) T2-weighted axial, after successful endoscopic fenestration. At presentation there is shift of midline structures and high intensity signal change in the white matter in the region of the trigone of the right lateral ventricle, indicating edema, presumably due to pressure (image A). These features settled after successful treatment (images B and C).

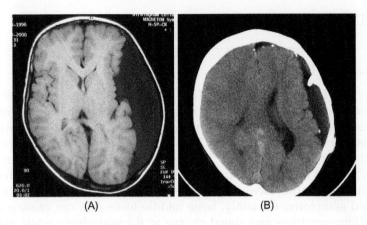

(A)   (B)

FIGURE 6.2   Radiological images of a 6-year-old child with persistent headaches and vomiting and a large left middle fossa AC, spreading over the convexity of the left cerebral hemisphere. (A) T1-weighted axial MR scan, at presentation. (B) CT scan after insertion of a cyst-peritoneal shunt. The large cyst is compressing the underlying hemisphere causing midline shift at presentation (image A). After successful treatment the midline shift has settled (image B).

Altered Cerebral Perfusion and Metabolism

It has been reported that ACs reduce perfusion and metabolism in surrounding cortical regions. These studies have been performed with the use of cerebral Single Photon Emission Computerized Tomography (SPECT) scan that uses isotopes to study rCBF (regional Cerebral Blood Flow). It is uncertain if the hypoperfusion is due to local compression of cerebral blood vessels by the cyst or due to a global effect of intracranial hypertension, because it has been observed even in vascular territories away from the cyst. Postoperative SPECT scans have shown normalization of rCBF after surgical cyst decompression [16,17]. The alteration in SPECT and rCBF can be used in decision making in relatively small or medium size cysts, although it is not regarded as a standard practice to perform SPECT scans in children routinely. The improvement of hypoperfusion is correlated to the improvement of the patient in neuropsychological testing and cognition [18–20].

Similar negative effect of ACs on cerebral metabolism has been reported. In patients with middle fossa cysts and language impairment and cognitive deficits, study of cerebral metabolism with ^{18}F fludeoxyglucose positron emission tomography (PET) scan demonstrated defects in cerebral metabolism, which improved after successful surgical cyst decompression, and this was correlated with clinical improvement of the cognitive defects [9] (Fig. 6.3).

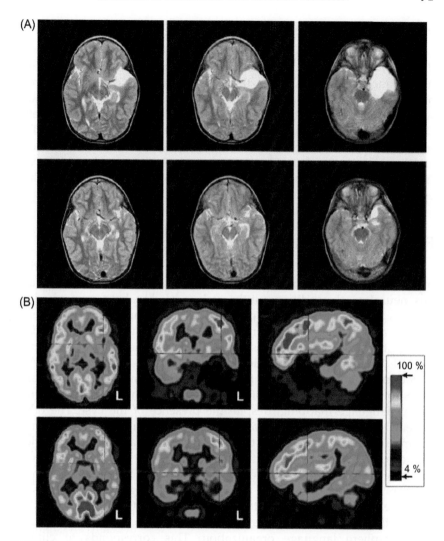

FIGURE 6.3 Effect of arachnoid cyst on cerebral metabolism. Radiological examinations of a patient with middle fossa arachnoid cyst and language and cognitive deficits, which improved after surgical treatment. (A) T2-weighted Axial MR scans before (upper row) and after (lower row) treatment. There is an arachnoid cyst in the left middle fossa which reduced drastically in size after cyst-peritoneal shunting, revealing healthy brain parenchyma underneath. (B) ^{18}F Fludeoxyglucose Positron Emission Tomography (PET) scans before (upper row) and after (lower row). There is hypometabolism in the cerebral parenchyma surrounding the arachnoid cyst (black area), which has improved significantly after cyst decompression, as judged by the presence of signal uptake in the parts of the brain where the cyst was previously. *Source: From Lai PH, Hsu SS, Ding SW, Ko CW, Ko CW, Fu JH, et al. Proton magnetic resonance spectroscopy and diffusion-weighted imaging in intracranial cystic mass lesions. Surg Neurol 2007;68 Suppl 1:S25-S36, with permission from Pediatric Neurology, Elsevier.*

MR Imaging Characteristics in DWI

Whilst in most cases the radiologic characteristics of ACs are clear, due to their CSF content, well demarcated rounded appearance, and nonenhancing walls, at times there is the need to differentiate from other cystic lesions, such as epidermoid cysts. The use of diffusion-weighted imaging (DWI) and measurement of apparent diffusion coefficient (ADC) values can be valuable in such circumstances. In DWI sequences epidermoid cysts (and other cystic lesions with proteinaceous and lipid content such as abscesses) have hyperintense signal whereas ACs have hypointense signal [21,22]. ACs have higher ADC values than epidermoid cysts [23].

Functional MR Imaging in ACs

Whilst fMRI has been used to investigate the functional organization of the cerebral cortex both in normal subjects and in patients with various neurological conditions, little such work has been performed in patients with ACs. One of the problems is the young age of the patients usually at diagnosis, which renders the application of paradigms difficult in the adverse conditions of an MR examination. A study performed in five asymptomatic patients with a left temporal AC, attempted to investigate the influence of the cyst in the cortical organization of language [24]. Four of these five patients had a clear left hemisphere language mapping, despite the presence of the cyst. The other patient had bilateral representation. What was interesting was the morphometric findings. Whilst in the left side there was decreased cortical thickness in association with the cyst, the surface area of the inferior frontal gyrus, which is regarded as the substrate for language, namely the pars triangularis and pars opercularis, was larger on the (left) side with the cyst, in comparison to the normal other (right) side. In other words, the presence of the cyst did not disturb the normal asymmetry of hemisphere language organization. This corresponds to clinical impressions, where children with temporal ACs are not found to have speech problems and their school performance is regarded normal, see also Chapter 6, Intracranial Arachnoid Cysts And Mental Functions, of Volume 2.

References

[1] Al-Holou WN, Yew AY, Boomsaad ZE, Garton HJ, Muraszko KM, Maher CO. Prevalence and natural history of arachnoid cysts in children. J Neurosurg Pediatr 2010;5(6):78–585.

[2] Morris Z, Whiteley WN, Longstreth Jr WT, Weber F, Lee YC, Tsushima Y, et al. Incidental findings on brain magnetic resonance imaging: systematic review and metaanalysis. BMJ 2009;339:b3016.

[3] Vernooij MW, Ikram MA, Tanghe HL, Vincent AJ, Hofman A, Krestin GP, et al. Incidental findings on brain MRI in the general population. N Engl J Med 2007;357:1821–8.

[4] Helland CA, Aarhus M, Knappskog P, Olsson L, Lund-Johansen M, Amiry-Moghaddam M, et al. Increased NKCC1 expression in arachnoid cysts supports secretory basis for cyst formation. Exp Neurol 2010;224:424–8.

[5] Tunes C, Flønes I, Helland C, Wilhemsen K, Goplen F, Wester KG. Pre- and post-operative dizziness and postural instability in temporal arachnoid cyst patients. Acta Neurol Scand 2014;129(5):335–42.

[6] Raveenthiran V, Reshma KB. Sixth cranial nerve palsy due to arachnoid cyst. J Pediatr Ophthalmol Strabismus 2014;51:e58–61 Online.

[7] Tarantino R, Marruzzo D, Colista D, Mancarella C, Delfini R. Twelfth nerve paresis induced by an unusual posterior fossa arachnoid cyst: case report and literature review. Br J Neurosurg 2014;28(4):528–30.

[8] Isaksen E, Leet TH, Helland CA, Wester K. Maze learning in patients with intracranial arachnoid cysts. Acta Neurochir (Wien) 2013;155(5):841–8.

[9] Laporte N, De Volder A, Bonnier C, Raftopoulos C, Sebire G. Language impairment associated with arachnoid cysts: recovery after surgical treatment. Pediatr Neurol 2012;46:44–7.

[10] Mørkve SH, Helland CA, Amus J, Lund-Johansen M, Wester KG. Surgical decompression of arachnoid cysts leads to improved quality of life: a prospective study. Neurosurgery 2016;78(5):613–25.

[11] Di Rocco C, Tamburrini G, Caldarelli M, Velardi F, Santini P. Prolonged ICP monitoring in Sylvian arachnoid cysts. Surg Neurol 2003;60(3):211–18.

[12] Germanò A, Caruso G, Caffo M, Baldari S, Calisto A, Meli F, et al. The treatment of large supratentorial arachnoid cysts in infants with cyst-peritoneal shunting and Hakim programmable valve. Childs Nerv Syst 2003;19(3):166–73.

[13] Helland CA, Wester K. Intracystic pressure in patients with temporal arachnoid cysts: a prospective study of preoperative complaints and postoperative outcome. J Neurol Neurosurg Psychiatry 2007;78(6):620–3.

[14] Baquero GA, Molero P, Pla J, Ortuno F. A schizophrenia-like psychotic disorder secondary to an arachnoid cyst remitted with neurosurgical treatment of the cyst. Open Neuroimag J 2014;8:1–4.

[15] Vidrih B, Karlovic D, Pasic MB. Arachnoid cyst as the cause of bipolar affective disorder: case report. Acta Clin Croat 2012;51(4):655–9.

[16] Martínez-Lage JF, Valentí JA, Piqueras C, Ruiz-Espejo AM, Román F, Nuño de la Rosa JA. Functional assessment of intracranial arachnoid cysts with TC99 m-HMPAO SPECT: a preliminary report. Childs Nerv Syst 2006;22(9):1091–7.

[17] Sgouros S, Chapman S. Congenital middle fossa arachnoid cysts may cause global brain ischaemia: a study with 99Tc-hexamethylpropyleneamineoxime single photon emission computerised tomography scans. Pediatr Neurosurg 2001;35(4):188–94.

[18] Gjerde PB, Schmid M, Hammar Å, Wester K. Intracranial arachnoid cysts: impairment of higher cognitive functions and postoperative improvement. J Neurodev Dis 2013;5:21.

[19] Raeder MB, Helland CA, Hugdahl K, Wester K. Arachnoid cysts cause cognitive deficits that improve after surgery. Neurology 2005;64:160–2.

[20] Soukup VM, Patterson J, Trier TT, Chen JW. Cognitive improvement despite minimal arachnoid cyst decompression. Brain Dev 1998;20:589–93.

[21] Lai PH, Hsu SS, Ding SW, Ko CW, Ko CW, Fu JH, et al. Proton magnetic resonance spectroscopy and diffusion-weighted imaging in intracranial cystic mass lesions. Surg Neurol 2007;68(Suppl. 1):S25−36.

[22] Bergui M, Zhong J, Bradac GB, Sales S. Diffusion-weighted images of intracranial cyst-like lesions. Neuroradiology 2001;43(10):824−9.

[23] Hakyemez B, Yildiz H, Ergin N, Uysal S, Parlak M. Flair and diffusion weighted MR imaging in differentiating epidermoid cysts from atachnoid cysts. Tani Girisim Radyol 2003;9(4):418−26 (Article in Turkish, abstract in English).

[24] Hund-Georgiadis M, Yves Von Cramon D, Kruggel F, Preul C. Do quiescent arachnoid cysts alter CNS functional organization? A fMRI and morphometric study. Neurology 2002;59(12):1935−9.

Biochemistry—Composition of and Possible Mechanisms for Production of Arachnoid Cyst Fluid

Magnus Berle[1,2] and Knut Wester[1,2]

[1]University of Bergen, Bergen, Norway
[2]Haukeland University Hospital, Bergen, Norway

OUTLINE

ABBREVIATIONS

AC   arachnoid cyst
ATPase   enzyme
CSF   cerebrospinal fluid
NKCC1   Na-K-Cl cotransporter 1

Arachnoid Cysts: Epidemiology, Biology, and Neuroimaging
DOI: http://dx.doi.org/10.1016/B978-0-12-809932-2.00007-7

BACKGROUND

Although arachnoid cysts (ACs) have been known for nearly two centuries [1], the mechanisms behind their formation are still uncertain. Several authors have evaluated the biochemistry and biology of ACs, however without reaching a definite conclusion as to their nature. As will be discussed below, analyzing the composition of cyst fluid may help shed light on these biological aspects of the cysts.

Starkman et al. in 1958 [2] observed that ACs are truly intraarachnoid in origin, a finding confirmed by electron microscopy by Rengachary et al. in 1978 [3]. The latter authors also performed a histopathological study including light, tramsmission, and scanning electron microscopic studies on four selected cases of AC [4], observing several structural features distinguishing AC membranes from normal arachnoid: the splitting of the arachnoid at the margin of the cyst; a thick layer of collagen in the wall; the absence of trabecular processes in the cyst; as well as hyperplastic arachnoid cells in the cyst wall. The collagen was believed to be reactive, as a consequence of pressure—clear arachnoid cells in the wall were suggested to be involved in the production of collagen. A striking feature of their article is the observation of an inner layer of the cyst membrane consisting of clear arachnoid cells. The authors described these clear arachnoid cells to be hypertrophic and hyperplastic with a resemblance to observed human fetal arachnoid cells. In the same publication [4], they also evaluated 208 previously reported cases of ACs and found that AC had a predilection for certain anatomical locations as there was a nearly invariable association of AC with normal subarachnoid cisterns; the most frequent location being the temporal fossa (49%). They suggested that AC develops as a congenital anomaly in the formation of subarachnoid cisterns.

Prior to the availability of CT, there was less systematic investigation of the prevalence of ACs; consequently ACs are mostly reported in case reports, relatively small patient series, selected age groups, or anatomical locations. However, there are also review articles based on these previous reports [5,6] and a few larger patient series [7,8]. By and large, it appears from these publications that the prevalence for the temporal fossa is higher than estimated by Rengachary and Watanabe [4]; nearly two-thirds are located there. The studies of ultrastructure and histopathology of ACs developed with the innovation of electron microscopes, giving the opportunity to properly examine the subcellular contents in layers of arachnoid membrane.

Starkman [2] suggested the splitting of the arachnoid membrane as a developmental artefact causing the formation of ACs, a view supported by Rengachary and coworkers [3,4]. Go et al. [9] reported the location of transport ATPase in the apical membrane of the ACs as an indication of a secretory function with a similarity to that of the choroid plexus.

There have been a multitude of theories on development largely based on case reports and smaller studies of individual material [1,2,10–12] without a certain conclusion. One of the authors (Wester) [13] suggested, on the basis of the observed predilection for the middle fossa as localization of AC, a mechanism that involved a defect in the early folding of the brain and meningeal anlage. Rabiei et al. [14] have recently published a large study on electron microscopic analyses on symptomatic cysts. They observed that of 24 cysts, only 12 had a structure that would be expected from an AC, see Chapter 5, Ultrastructure of Arachnoid Cysts. This finding is in particular worth observing for the design of new explorative studies, in particular with respect to our own studies of cyst fluid [15,16]. The authors believe that analyses of AC fluid can give an indication to the mechanisms of filling and to the sustaining of the cysts.

THEORIES OF FILLING MECHANISM

There are three prevailing theories on the mechanisms of filling and sustaining of such cysts [17]; active pumps, a valve mechanism, or oncotic pressure. Go et al. [9] suggested a mechanism of fluid secretion based on cytochemical identification of an active pump in the cyst membrane, more precisely transport ATPase in the luminal surface membrane. Dyck and Gruskin [18] suggested that osmotic pressure gradients were involved in the filling of the cysts, as also implied by Schachenmayr and Friede [19]. Smith and Smith [20], later supported by among others Santamarta et al. [21], have suggested several types of one-way valves as a mechanism by which fluid enters the cyst. Secondary ACs develop as a result of head injury, meningitis, or tumors, or as a complication of brain surgery [22]. We do not know of separate cyst fluid studies exploring the subject (Text Box 7.1).

BIOCHEMICAL STUDIES

Concerning the fluid content of ACs, Sandberg et al. [23] examined the content of pediatric ACs, finding a liquid comparable to cerebrospinal fluid (CSF) reference in chemical content and osmotic pressure. Some of the reported cysts had elevated protein content, not fully explained by the authors. The authors pointed to the lack of control material as a limitation of their study.

TEXT BOX 7.1

SUGGESTED MECHANISMS FOR PRODUCTION OF ARACHNOID CYST FLUID

Active transport is a pump mechanism in the membrane of the cyst creating a pressure upholding the cyst.

Osmotic pressure gradients imply an influx of water because of an osmotic active content of the cyst.

One-way valve mechanisms suggest a trapping of liquid, probably CSF, in the cyst.

Secondary cysts are suggested as a different entity, possible due to inflammatory processes after a trauma.

In one of our own studies [16], we sampled AC fluid and CSF intraoperatively in 15 patients with temporal cysts. Before the craniotomy, a small burr hole was made immediately posterior to the sphenoid wing in order to gain access to the anterior and most basal aspects of the middle cranial fossa, allowing the underlying dura and cyst membrane to be punctured and cyst fluid to be sampled before opening the dura. CSF was collected from the prepontine subarachnoid space after cyst fenestration and the molecular composition of the two fluids were compared. The collection of AC fluid and CSF is illustrated in Fig. 7.1. We found a chemical composition of the cyst fluid that resembled CSF, however, some proteins (albumin, lactate dehydrogenase, and ferritin)

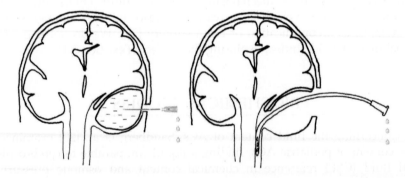

FIGURE 7.1 Illustration of sampling method of arachnoid cyst fluid through a syringe needle and collection of CSF from the prepontine subarachnoid space through a baby feeding tube.

in general had a lower concentration in AC fluid than in CSF—the data from the publication presented in Table 7.1. We observed that the osmolarity and the concentration of salt molecules in AC fluid and CSF is very similar. These findings seem to be in line with the findings of Sandberg et al. [23]—data presented in Table 7.2. On the other side, Sandberg et al. found an elevated protein content in the AC fluid based on estimated values.

The conclusions we drew from our studies were (1) we did not identify a plausible driving mechanism for the osmotic pressure in the AC, thus our data do not support an osmotic mechanism. We do not observe a difference in osmolarity, but this sort of osmolarity difference would be not likely to be observed, as water can flow relatively freely over cell

TABLE 7.1   Data From Chemical Analyses of AC Fluid by Berle et al.

Analysis	Unit	n	Mean AC Fluid +/− SEM	Mean CSF Fluid +/− SEM	Mean Cyst/CSF
Sodium	mmol/L	13	142.23 +/− 2.14	142.08 +/− 2.71	1.00
Potassium	mmol/L	13	2.47 +/− 0.04	2.35 +/− 0.07	1.05
Chloride	mmol/L	13	121.23 +/− 1.94	120.15 +/− 2.54	1.01
Calcium	mmol/L	13	1.07 +/− 0.01	1.03 +/− 0.03	1.04
Magnesium	mmol/L	13	1.20 +/− 0.01	1.14 +/− 0.03	1.05
Phosphate	mmol/L	13	0.39 +/− 0.01	0.35 +/− 0.01	1.11*
Glucose	mmol/L	13	2.85 +/− 0.09	3.13 +/− 0.11	0.92
Protein	g/L	13	0.30 +/− 0.03	0.41 +/− 0.04	0.71**
Lactate dehydrogenase	U/L	13	17.91 +/− 2.93	35.55 +/− 4.61	0.57**
Ferritin	ug/L	13	7.82 +/− 1.00	25.55 +/− 6.20	0.31**
Osmolarity	mosmol/L	13	290.15 +/− 1.07	290.08 +/− 0.96	1
IgG	g/L		<1.50	<1.50	
IgA	g/L		<0.25	<0.25	
IgM	g/L		<0.18	<0.18	
Iron	umol/L		Low	Low	
Triglycerides	mmol/L		Low	Low	

Data from Berle M, Wester KG, Ulvik RJ, Kroksveen AC, Haaland OA, Amiry-Moghaddam M, et al. Arachnoid cysts do not contain cerebrospinal fluid: a comparative chemical analysis of arachnoid cyst fluid and cerebrospinal fluid in adults. Cerebrospinal Fluid Res 2010;7(1), 8. http://dx.doi.org/10.1743-8454-7-8 [pii] 10.1186/1743-8454-7-8 showing the biochemical composition of AC fluid and CSF.

TABLE 7.2   Data From Chemical Analyses of AC Fluid by Berle et al.

Analysis	Unit	n	Range	Median	Mean	EV
protein	mg/dL	41	9.0–3100.0	37.0	178.2	25.6
sodium	mEq/L	38	136.0–159.0	140.0	142.2	143.3
potassium	mEq/L	17	2.4–3.7	2.6	2.7	2.9
chloride	mEq/L	26	113.0–125.0	122.0	120.8	120.3
osmolarity	mOsm/kg	35	277.0–335.0	284.0	285.5	287.2
glucose	mg/dL	37	26.0–98.0	51.0	53.2	NA
WBC	count/mm^3	44	0.0–410.0	1.0	NA	NA
RBC	count/mm^3	44	0.0–100,000.0	1.5	NA	NA

Data from Sandberg DI, McComb JG, Krieger MD. Chemical analysis of fluid obtained from intracranial arachnoid cysts in pediatric patients. J Neurosurg 2005;103(5 Suppl), 427–432. doi:10.3171/ ped.2005.103.5.0427 showing the biochemical composition of AC fluid versus estimated values.

membranes. (2) If there were a slit valve, we would expect the molecules of CSF to flow freely through a slit valve, but not of that of an active transport mechanism due to selectivity of transport or molecule size. This made us conclude that these findings did not support a slit valve.

We followed up the previous study by quantitative proteomics of the cyst fluid versus CSF from the same patients [15]. The objective of this study was by using proteomics to look for cues to a possible mechanism. The biochemical studies performed earlier examined only three proteins; we intended to perform a more thorough examination of the same material. We identified significant differences in quantity of proteins between the sample materials (AC fluid and CSF), but we were not able to interpret with certainty the mechanisms behind these differences. We did observe [16] that two of the cysts could be secondary cysts by the patient's medical history. These two patients had a very elevated protein content.

We have reflected on limitations of the strategy of fluid sampling. First, that contamination of blood/plasma could alter the expression of protein. As the concentration of protein in blood is 100–200 times higher than that of CSF, results are prone to error due to contamination. Secondly, due to ethics and technical feasibility, there is no easy way to obtain either sample material or an adequate control. We do not know of a better way to examine the cyst fluid than our chosen method. Thirdly, if a possible mechanism is cellular or membrane-bound, there is no certainty that this mechanism will be detectable by a liquid sampling strategy. The suspected pump mechanisms, the ATPases, identified by Go and coworkers [9], would be difficult to detect with such a strategy. To date, this is the largest study of AC fluid.

Rabiei and coworkers [14] demonstrated a heterogeneity in the lining of the AC. This opens up a discussion of whether ACs might be more than one condition.

OSMOTIC PRESSURE MECHANISM

The osmotic pressure mechanism suggests that the content of the cysts have a high oncotic pressure, thus attracting water and creating a pressure on the walls of the cyst. This would be a gradual process leading to cyst expansion. Such a mechanism would normally be an elevated albumin or other macromolecule inside the cyst. Albumin in the blood circulation is a negatively charged macromolecule. Briefly, this negative charge attracts positive ions of salts as electrolytes thus creating the oncotic pressure binding water. The expected finding would be an elevated protein content. Oncotic pressure mechanisms would attract water instantly in the body; we would not expect to see any change in the osmotic pressure. The two studies [16,23] of the chemical composition of AC fluid do not support osmosis as a single driver of cyst growth, because of the lack of a source to drive the osmotic pressure. The protein content in the AC fluid examined by Sandberg et al. [23] showed a large variability in protein content, and thus less consistent with this as a single driver of osmotic pressure. Our own study [16] revealed a reduced protein content in AC fluid versus CSF from the same patient, although that was with the limitations with the sampling of the CSF. In secondary cysts, the protein concentration is elevated and oncotic pressure mechanisms might be a part of this subgroup of cysts.

VALVE MECHANISM

A number of publications have reported the observation of a unidirectional valve either perioperatively or by neuroimaging. [10,21,24−29], but the observations are limited to the suprasellar or parasellar region. The valve mechanism has not been studied properly from a biochemical viewpoint. One would intuitively expect that a larger slit valve that allows CSF to enter a preformed cavity and thus build up an increased pressure would result in a similar biochemical composition of the cyst fluid and CSF. As opposed to a valve mechanism, passive pores would not by the same intuition let the pressure build up to cause formation of cysts—such a mechanism seems again less intuitive.

ACTIVE TRANSPORT

An active transport or secretion mechanism might cause a chemical change that is detectable in the cyst fluid. This might be a mechanism of transcytosis, where vesicula of content are transported through the lining cells or salt pumps creating a gradient of oncotic pressure attracting water. Go et al. have demonstrated that the morphological features of the cells lining AC are consistent with fluid secretion capacity [9,30,31]. There are a variety of mechanisms in the body that might be involved, but none are currently proved. The biochemical composition of the cyst fluid would necessarily be dependent on the filling mechanism. Due to sampling difficulties of both cyst fluid and normal control, this might be challenging to detect. A perspective worth noting is the placement of salt pumps, necessarily being membrane-bound. Such pumps would have to be nonwater soluble as a part of the lipid membrane. Proteomics of the water compartment is not necessarily a strategy that can detect such pumps. Go et al. [9] demonstrated a structural organization of a Na^+K^+ ATPase indication fluid transport towards the lumen. Helland et al. [32] identified upregulation of the $Na^+K^+2Cl^-$ cotransporter $NKCC1^-$ gene in AC membrane when compared with normal arachnoid membrane. We conclude that for primary ACs, an active mechanism for filling seems to be the probable cause, but further research is needed.

References

[1] Bright R. Reports of Medical Cases, selected with a view of illustration the symptoms and cure of Diseases, by a reference to Morbid Anatomy. Diseases of the Brain and Nervous System, part II, vol. II. London: Longman; 1827-31. p. 538 Rees, Orme, Brown & Green.

[2] Starkman SP, Brown TC, Linell EA. Cerebral arachnoid cysts. J Neuropathol Exp Neurol 1958;17(3):484−500.

[3] Rengachary SS, Watanabe I, Brackett CE. Pathogenesis of intracranial arachnoid cysts. Surg Neurol 1978;9(2):139−44.

[4] Rengachary SS, Watanabe I. Ultrastructure and pathogenesis of intracranial arachnoid cysts. J Neuropathol Exp Neurol 1981;40(1):61−83.

[5] Gosalakkal JA. Intracranial arachnoid cysts in children: a review of pathogenesis, clinical features, and management. Pediatr Neurol 2002;26:93−8.

[6] Wester K. Gender distribution and sidedness of middle fossa arachnoid cysts: a review of cases diagnosed with computer imaging. Neurosurgery 1992;31:940−4.

[7] Helland CA, Lund-Johansen M, Wester K. Location, sidedness, and sex distribution of intracranial arachnoid cysts in a population-based sample. J Neurosurg 2010;113 (5):934−9. Available from: http://dx.doi.org/10.3171/2009.11.JNS081663.

[8] Sakai N, Kumagai M, Ueda T, Iwamura M, Nishimura Y, Miwa Y, et al. Clinical study on intracranial arachnoid cyst: with reference to the middle cranial fossa. No Shinkei Geka 1989;17:117−23.

[9] Go KG, Houthoff HJ, Blaauw EH, Havinga P, Hartsuiker J. Arachnoid cysts of the sylvian fissure. Evidence of fluid secretion. J Neurosurg 1984;60(4):803–13. Available from: http://dx.doi.org/10.3171/jns.1984.60.4.0803.

[10] Hornig GW, Zervas NT. Slit defect og the diaphragma sellae with valve effect: observation of a "slit valve". Neurosurgery 1992;30:265–7.

[11] Jakubiak P, Dunsmore RH, Beckett RS. Supratentorial brain cysts. J Neurosurg 1968;28:129–36.

[12] Robinson RG. The temporal lobe agenesis syndrome. Brain 1964;87:87–106 PMID: 14152215.

[13] Wester K. Peculiarities of intracranial arachnoid cysts: location, sidedness, and sex distribution in 126 consecutive patients. Neurosurgery 1999;45(4):775–9.

[14] Rabiei K, Tisell M, Wikkelsø C, Johansson B. Diverse arachnoid cyst morphology indicates different pathophysiological origins. Fluids Barriers CNS 2014;11(5):1–11. Available from: http://dx.doi.org/10.1186/2045-8118-11-5.

[15] Berle M, Kroksveen AC, Garberg H, Aarhus M, Haaland OA, Wester K, et al. Quantitative proteomics comparison of arachnoid cyst fluid and cerebrospinal fluid collected perioperatively from arachnoid cyst patients. Fluids Barriers CNS 2013;10 (1):17. Available from: http://dx.doi.org/10.1186/2045-8118-10-17.

[16] Berle M, Wester KG, Ulvik RJ, Kroksveen AC, Haaland OA, Amiry-Moghaddam M, et al. Arachnoid cysts do not contain cerebrospinal fluid: a comparative chemical analysis of arachnoid cyst fluid and cerebrospinal fluid in adults. Cerebrospinal Fluid Res 2010;7(1):8 http://dx.doi.org/10.1743-8454-7-8 [pii] 10.1186/1743-8454-7-8.

[17] Cincu R, Agrawal A, Eiras J. Intracranial arachnoid cysts: current concepts and treatment alternatives. Clin Neurol Neurosurg 2007;109(10):837–43 http://dx.doi.org/10. S0303-8467(07)00193-X [pii]. http://dx.doi.org/10.1016/j.clineuro.2007.07.013.

[18] Dyck P, Gruskin P. Supratentorial arachnoid cysts in adults. A discussion of two cases from a pathophysiologic and surgical perspective. Arch Neurol 1977;34(5): 276–9.

[19] Schachenmayr W, Friede RL. Fine structure of arachnoid cysts. J Neuropathol Exp Neurol 1979;38(4):434–46.

[20] Smith RA, Smith WA. Arachnoid cysts of the middle cranial fossa. Surg Neurol 1976;5(4):246–52.

[21] Santamarta D, Aguas J, Ferrer E. The natural history of arachnoid cysts: endoscopic and cine-mode MRI evidence of a slit-valve mechanism. Minim Invasive Neurosurg 1995;38(4):133–7. Available from: http://dx.doi.org/10.1055/s-2008-1053473.

[22] NINDS. NINDS Arachnoid Cysts Information Page. Retrieved from http://www. ninds.nih.gov/disorders/arachnoid_cysts/arachnoid_cysts.htm.

[23] Sandberg DI, McComb JG, Krieger MD. Chemical analysis of fluid obtained from intracranial arachnoid cysts in pediatric patients. J Neurosurg 2005;103(Suppl. 5):427–32. Available from: http://dx.doi.org/10.3171/ped.2005.103.5.0427.

[24] Al-Din AN, Williams B. A case of high-pressure intracerebral pouch. J Neurol Neurosurg Psychiatry 1981;44:918–23.

[25] Koga H, Mukawa J, Miyagi K, Kinjo T, Okuyama K. Symptomatic intraventricular arachnoid cyst in an elderly man. Acta Neurochir (Wien) 1995;137:113–17.

[26] Kumagai M, Sakai N, Yamada H, Shinoda J, Nakashima T, Iwama T, et al. Postnatal development and enlargement of primary middle cranial fossa arachnoid cyst recognized on repeat CT scans. Childs Nerv Syst 1986;2:211–15.

[27] Schroeder HW, Gaab MR. Endoscopic observation of a slit-valve mechanism in a suprasellar prepontine arachnoid cyst: case report. Neurosurgery 1997;40:198–200.

[28] Caemaert J, Abdullah J, Calliauw L, Carton D, Dhooge C, van Coster R. Endoscopic treatment of suprasellar arachnoid cysts. Acta Neurochir (Wien) 1992;119 (1–4):68–73.

[29] Choi JU, Kim DS, Huh R. Endoscopic approach to arachnoid cyst. Childs Nerv Syst
      1999;15:285−91.
[30] Go KG, Houthoff HJ, Blaauw EH, Stokroos I, Blauuw G. Scanning and transmission
      electron microscopy of three cases. Acta Neuropathol (Berl) 1978;44:57−62.
[31] Go KG, Houthoff HJ, Hartsuiker J, Blaauw EH, Havinga P. Fluid secretion in arach-
      noid cysts as a clue to cerebrospinal fluid absorption at the arachnoid granulation.
      J Neurosurg 1986;65:642−8.
[32] Helland CA, Aarhus M, Knappskog P, Olsson LK, Lund-Johansen M, Amiry-
      Moghaddam M, et al. Increased NKCC1 expression in arachnoid cysts supports
      secretory basis for cyst formation. Exp Neurol 2010; http://dx.doi.org/10.S0014-4886
      (10)00160-3 [pii] 10.1016/j.expneurol.2010.05.002.

The "Valve Mechanism"

David Santamarta and Emilio González-Martínez
University Hospital of León, León, Spain

ABBREVIATIONS

BA basilar artery
CSF cerebrospinal fluid
MR magnetic resonance
P Pons

RECOMMENDATIONS—LEVEL OF EVIDENCE

Levels I–III

There is no level I–III evidence available for topics covered in this chapter.

Level IV

There is only level IV evidence available for topics covered in this chapter.

INTRODUCTION

It is widely accepted that arachnoid cysts result from abnormal embryologic development of the arachnoid and the subarachnoid space with secondary displacement of the brain [1,2]. However, the mechanism by which arachnoid cysts fill up and achieve an expansive behavior is one of the most contentious issues.

Over time, three theories have prevailed: active secretion of fluid by cells in the cyst wall; fluid influx due to an osmotic pressure gradient; and trapping of fluid by what has somehow been misleadingly termed a "valve mechanism" [2–4]. A main consideration related to this latter argument is how the fluid enters and exits the cystic cavity. The concern regarding arachnoid cysts comes from the inability of cerebrospinal fluid (CSF) to freely flow throughout the subarachnoid space and cisterns. CSF circulation appears to play an essential role in the pathophysiology of arachnoid cysts.

This chapter is devoted to upholding the so-called "valve mechanism," providing justification for its pathophysiological hypothesis, but also discussing the main limitations of this model.

HISTORICAL BACKGROUND

Williams and Guthkelch, in elucidating the pathogenesis of arachnoid cysts, suggested the possibility of imperceptible communications between the cyst and CSF pathways. They proposed the primary driving force behind CSF flow and eventual enlargement of arachnoid cysts was a pulsatile pump mechanism [5]. Some years later, different authors spread the use of cisternography with metrizamide and computed tomographic scanning to address the issue of inadequate communication between the cyst and the subarachnoid space. From those studies a classification scheme for Sylvian fissure cysts emerged, in which there is an inverse relationship between the existence and degree of communication and the size and mass effect of the cyst [6]. Therefore, arachnoid cysts have been widely regarded as communicating or noncommunicating, see also Chapter 10, Classification and Location of Arachnoid Cysts.

Although the existence of a *slit-valve mechanism* had been theoretically proposed, Caemaert first reported it in a suprasellar arachnoid cyst [7]. Since then, a valve mechanism has been frequently described, but never in other locations.

COMMUNICATION WITH SUBARACHNOID SPACE

Arachnoid cysts behave as entrapped collections of fluid variably communicating with the subarachnoid space [8]. Most cysts remain stable in size and rarely disappear, demonstrating that secretion is neither universal nor the only mechanism involved. Moreover, there has been no direct evidence of fluid production within the cyst. Indirect morphological features supporting active fluid transport have led to this hypothesis [4]. Data coming from accumulation of fluid by an osmotic pressure gradient are scarce and impractical from a clinical standpoint, see Chapter 7, Biochemistry—Composition of and Possible Mechanisms for Production of Arachnoid Cyst Fluid.

Some of them may have a patent and free communication with adjoining cisterns. By contrast, it is hard to demonstrate a tiny or free passage of fluid between the cyst and the subarachnoid space in others, regardless of the method used to investigate an eventual communication (flow-sensitive magnetic resonance (MR) sequences, contrast agents, or intraoperative endoscopic inspection). Whatever the nature of this communication, be it virtual or patent, most importantly fluid is not stagnant inside the cyst, but seems to flows throughout it (Fig. 8.1). This assumption has been observed by modern radiological techniques such as phase-contrast cine MR. Up to 30% of arachnoid cysts present communication with subarachnoid space [9].

Neuroimaging studies play a crucial role in accurately diagnosing arachnoid cysts. High-resolution MR sequences delineate the membranous borders of the cyst, and therefore define the anatomical boundaries sharply. MR also provides a functional complement to anatomic imaging for the investigation of arachnoid cysts due to its sensitivity to moving fluid.

Fluid flow is difficult to study in living systems. An appropriate technology to measure and model flowing CSF or the behavior of fluid under physiological conditions is under development and has not

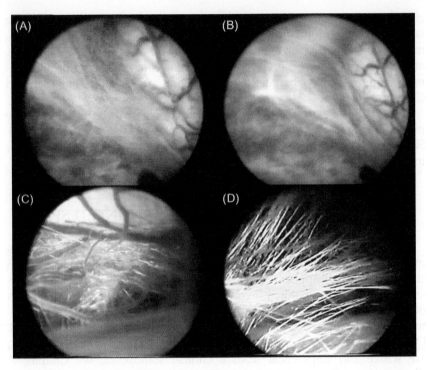

FIGURE 8.1 Different aspects of the arachnoid wall in a sylvian arachnoid cyst obtained with an endoscope within the cavity. In some areas it is a milky and tough veil (A), while in others the wall has a looser reticular appearance (C, D). At a certain phase of the cardiac cycle the arachnoid detaches from the solid surfaces (A) or merges with them (B).

reached widespread use [10]. The ideal goal would be to make flow visible without disturbing it. We need to see the grain in the stone.

Functional imaging with flow-sensitive MR sequences suggests different patterns of CSF flow within the cystic cavity [11]. One of these patterns points to a well-defined communication (*flow entry zone*) between the cyst and the subarachnoid space (Fig. 8.2). The *flow entry zone* is characterized by an area of low signal intensity, which indicates rapidly flowing CSF. Arachnoid maldevelopment and ineffective communication between the cyst and the subarachnoid space are involved in the pathophysiology of arachnoid cysts [8]. The consequences of defective CSF circulation may be so subtle than they can be easily overlooked or even ignored. Absence of an apparent *flow entry zone* does not necessarily mean isolation. The actual site or sites of communication may not always be evident because the magnitude of the flow may be below the detection sensitivity of the pulsing sequence or it may not lie within the imaged section.

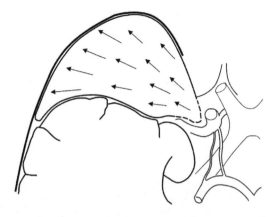

FIGURE 8.2   The draw illustrates a temporal arachnoid cyst. Its medial wall variably communicates with the basal cisterns, either through a patent *flow entry zone* or through tiny perforations.

"SLIT-VALVE MECHANISM"

Apart from the existence of communication between arachnoid cysts and subarachnoid space, another functional anatomic feature is the occasional visualization of a slit in the arachnoid acting as a "valve mechanism" in suprasellar arachnoid cysts [3,7,12]. This arachnoid sheet usually lies close to a major artery and a cistern (Fig. 8.3). The slit opens and closes during the cardiac cycle enabling fluid to fill and flush the cyst.

Some findings support this one-way configuration: the detection of a jet-like CSF flow into the suprasellar arachnoid cyst through cine-phase contrast MRI [3] and the presence of debris inside the cyst originating from the ventriculocystostomy procedure [12].

The primary driving force behind CSF flow and eventual enlargement of arachnoid cysts has stimulated debate. It is traditionally assumed that the arterial pulse conducts the energy, acting as the pump especially if closely surrounded by arachnoid adhesion [13]. Sudden contraction of the artery pulls the arachnoid attached to it, but the movement of the arachnoid itself is not so impetuous. There is an interval within the cardiac cycle in which the slit remains open. Hence, during this interval, fluid moves conceivably following a pressure gradient. However, only momentarily and when extracystic pressure overcomes intracystic pressure, CSF flows into the cyst, leading to the expansion of the arachnoid cyst. The arterial inflow has been considered inefficient to mediate a pump-like mechanism after having observed that the intracranial arterial diameter scarcely increases during systole.

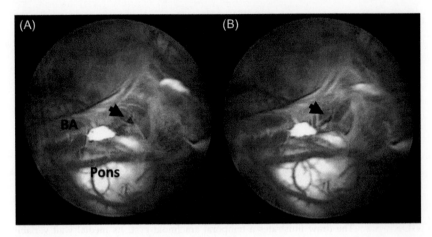

FIGURE 8.3 Images of the *slit-valve mechanism* obtained with an endoscope from a right precoronal approach. The slit (arrow) in the arachnoid next to the basilar artery opens during arterial inflow (A) and closes during basilar contraction (B). There is an interval in which the slit remains open allowing movement of CSF according to a pressure gradient. *BA*, basilar artery; *P*, pons.

Williams and Guthkelch emphasized the sensitivity of the subarachnoid space to changes in venous pressure [5]. Transient pressure gradients and a relatively larger amount of volume of CSF displaced during Valsalva maneuvers than during the cardiac cycle render the venous route a pathogenic factor implied in the expansive behavior of arachnoid cysts.

Whether by arterial or venous mechanism, these functional features support the existence of an anatomical communication between the subarachnoid space and the cyst. The arachnoid sheet itself is the barrier to freely flowing CSF. The communication, either as pores or slits, behaves functionally as a valve retarding and directing the flow of CSF. Transitory increases in pressure (i.e., arterial inflow during the cardiac cycle or Valsalva maneuvers) would ensure the gradients driving CSF to fill and flush the arachnoid cyst.

On the other hand, it has also been argued that Valsalva maneuvers can produce sufficient force to tear the arachnoid accelerating a natural decompression [14]. This favorable outcome focuses on the pathophysiology of arachnoid cysts on an altered pattern of CSF dynamics within the cyst due to hindered communication between the cystic cavity and the subarachnoid space.

Arachnoid maldevelopment and pulsatile CSF flow during each cardiac cycle leads to a gradual enlargement of the cyst. Accordingly, symptomatic cysts of suprasellar location have been mainly reported in childhood [15]. On the other hand, a natural decompression throughout the early years of life may be more common than is suggested in literature, since systematic surveillance of asymptomatic cases is lacking.

CONTROVERSIES

Although the *slit-valve mechanism* is the most appealing and elemental theory to explain the enlargement of arachnoid cysts, this pragmatism is controversial, and subject to discussion. It has been reported only in suprasellar arachnoid cysts, and any study has identified neither radiological nor endoscopical observations in other locations [15].

Regardless of location, arachnoid cysts seem to behave similarly: they result from a developmental abnormality in the arachnoid membrane; frequently they are discovered incidentally; and most arachnoid cysts are quiescent and remain stable throughout life. From the requirement to explain these similarities emerges the necessity of determining a unified theory. The *slit-valve mechanism* does not satisfy it since it has been only observed, as aforementioned, in suprasellar arachnoid cysts.

Some authors have based their arguments for supporting the *slit-valve mechanism* on the similarities described between CSF within and without the cyst. Although intra- and extracavitary components of arachnoid cysts have been defined as similar, ultrastructural analyses reveal that these differences are not minor. Current studies have emphasized protein concentration differences between intracystic and extracystic CSF. Reduced protein content in arachnoid cyst relative to CSF seems to override hypotheses such as the oncotic gradient or *slit-valve mechanism* [16,17]. Accordingly, as CSF composition is not exactly the same, it has been suggested to use the term "CSF-like fluid" instead of CSF in arachnoid cysts [16]. Go et al. observed the presence of microvilli on the luminal surface and cytoplasmic vesicles, and the existence of choroid plexus ectopia inside a growing arachnoid cyst has been reported [4,18]. Therefore, there is morphological and ultrastructural evidence to support the secretory nature of the cyst wall.

However, all these findings have been observed in temporal arachnoid cysts, and it is bias to extrapolate them to the whole entity. Even more so if the diversity of arachnoid cyst morphology is taken into account. Raibei et al. described three patterns: cysts composed of arachnoid-like tissue; cysts composed of fibrous connective tissue; and cysts with aberrant structure [1], see Chapter 5, Ultrastructure of Arachnoid Cysts. This would indicate that arachnoid cysts represent a heterogeneous group of pathological conditions and, presumably, different pathophysiological enlargement mechanisms. Therefore, the presence of a *slit-valvemechanism* in suprasellar arachnoid cysts does not exclude the secretary process of the cyst wall in arachnoid cysts in other locations.

References

[1] Rabiei K, Tisell M, Johansson BR. Diverse arachnoid cyst morphology indicates different pathophysiological origins. Fluids Barriers CNS 2014;11(1):5.

[2] Basaldella L, Orvieto E, Longatti P. Causes of arachnoid cyst development and expansion. Neurosurg Focus 2007;22(2):E4.

[3] Santamarta D, Aguas J, Ferrer E. The natural history of arachnoid cysts. Endoscopic and cine-mode MRI evidence of a slit-valve mechanism. Minim Invas Neurosurg 1995;38:133–7.

[4] Go KG, Houthoff EH, Hartsuiker J. Arachnoid cysts of the sylvian fissure. Evidence of fluid secretion. J Neurosurg 1984;60:803–13.

[5] Williams B, Guthkelch AN. Why do central arachnoid pouches expand? J Neurol Neurosurg Psych 1974;37:1085–92.

[6] Galassi E, Tognetti F, Frank G. CT scan and metrizamide CT cisternography in arachnoid cysts of the middle cranial fossa: classification and pathophysiological aspects. Surg Neurol 1982;17:363–9.

[7] Caemaert J, Abdullah J, van Coster R. Endoscopic treatment of suprasellar arachnoid cysts. Acta Neurochir 1992;119:68–73.

[8] Santamarta D, Morales F, Sierra JM, de Campos JM. Arachnoid cysts: entrapped collections of cerebrospinal fluid variably communicating with the subarachnoid space. Minim Invas Neurosurg 2001;44:128–34.

[9] Yildiz H, Erdogan C, Tuncel E. Evaluation of communication between intracranial arachnoid cysts and cisterns with phase-contrast cine MR imaging. AJNR Am J Neuroradiol 2005;26(1):145–51.

[10] Balédent O, Gondry-Jouet C, Meyer ME. Value of phase contrast magnetic resonance imaging for investigation of cerebral hydrodynamics. J Neuroradiol 2006;33:292–303.

[11] Hoffmann KT, Hosten N, Meyer BU, Röricht S, Sprung C, Oellinger J, Gutberlet M, Felix R. CSF flow studies of intracranial cysts and cyst-like lesions achieved using reversed fast imaging with steady-state precession MR sequences. AJNR Am J Neuroradiol 2000;21:493–502.

[12] Schroeder HW, Gaab MR. Endoscopic observation of a slit-valve mechanism in a suprasellar prepontine arachnoid cyst: case report. Neurosurgery 1997;40:198–200.

[13] Dott NM, Gillingham FJ. Mechanical aspects of the cerebrospinal fluid circulation-physiological, pathological, surgical. Ciba Found Symp Cereb Fluid 1958;246–60.

[14] Bristol RE, Albuquerque FC, Spetzler RE. Arachnoid cysts: spontaneous resolution distinct from traumatic rupture. Neurosurg Focus 2007;22(2):E2.

[15] Halani SH, Safain MG, Heilman CB. Arachnoid cyst slit valves: the mechanism for arachnoid cyst enlargement. J Neurosurg Pediatr 2013;12(1):62–6.

[16] Berle M, Wester KG, Helland CA. Arachnoid cysts do not contain cerebrospinal fluid: a comparative chemical analysis of arachnoid cyst fluid and cerebrospinal fluid in adults. Cerebrospinal Fluid Res 2010;10(7):8.

[17] Berle M, Kroksveen AC, Berven F. Quantitative proteomics comparison of arachnoid cyst fluid and cerebrospinal fluid collected perioperatively from arachnoid cyst patients. Fluids Barriers CNS 2013;10(1):17.

[18] Schuhmann MU, Tatagiba M, Samii M. Ectopic choroid plexus within a juvenile arachnoid cyst of the cerebellopontine angle: cause of cyst formation or reason of cyst growth. Pediatr Neurosurg 2000;32:73–6.

PREVALENCE AND NATURAL HISTORY OF ARACHNOID CYSTS

9

The Prevalence of Intracranial Arachnoid Cysts

Frank Weber

German Air Force Center of Aerospace Medicine, Fuerstenfeldbruck, Germany

ABBREVIATIONS

AC	arachnoid cyst
CSF	cerebrospinal fluid
CT	computerized tomography
HUNT	a large population-based health survey in a Norwegian county
MRI	magnetic resonance imaging

Arachnoid cysts (ACs) are fluid-filled malformations of the arachnoid tissue. Congenital, genetic, and traumatic factors have been suggested as the underlying mechanisms [1]. ACs usually arise within and expand the margins of cerebrospinal fluid (CSF) cisterns rich in arachnoid, i.e., Sylvian fissure, suprasellar, quadrigeminal, cerebellopontine angle, and posterior infratentorial midline cisterns. Congenital ACs are maldevelopmental anomalies in which splitting or duplication of the primitive arachnoid membrane in the early embryonal life leads to the collection of clear CSF-like fluid. This can be accompanied by atrophy of the adjacent cerebral tissue or can cause a mass effect. The majority of the ACs remain clinically silent throughout the individual's lifetime. If ACs become symptomatic, this occurs usually in regions where a mass effect becomes clinically evident early in the course of the expansion, i.e., in the sellar or suprasellar region [2].

Disease prevalence is an important measure of the burden of disease. ACs are frequent findings on intracranial imaging, however, their prevalence is not well defined. With the increasing use of neuroimaging (CT and MRI) there has been a corresponding increase in the number of incidentally reported ACs. I am now going to review a series of papers specifically designed to detect ACs or other incidental findings.

The first large study on the prevalence of ACs was performed by Becker and colleagues [3]. They examined a sample of 27,187 CT-scans and found a prevalence of ACs of 0.32%. Their sample was hospital-based patients that were recruited from a single university medical center. In 2006, Weber and Knopf reported a MRI study on incidental findings and found a prevalence of ACs of 1.80%. Their sample was highly selected and was composed of healthy young men who applied for the flying service in the German military [4]. The Rotterdam study was conducted to determine the prevalence of incidental findings in the general population [5]. ACs were found with a prevalence of 1.10% out of 2000 MRI scans. Kumar et al. published an MRI study on the prevalence of structural brain abnormalities in asymptomatic individuals and evaluated a random sample of 60–64-year-old community-dwelling individuals [6]. They reported two ACs in 478 individuals (prevalence 0.42%). Morris and colleagues reported in a systematic review and meta-analysis on incidental findings on brain magnetic resonance imaging [7]. In terms of ACs, this review was based on 15,559 individuals (total $n = 19,559$), a prevalence of 0.50% was described. ACs were the single most prevalent incidental finding in this investigation. One year later, Al-Holou reviewed a consecutive series of 11,738 children (i.e., persons younger than 18 years) who had undergone brain MRI at the university of Michigan health system between 1997 and 2008 for ACs and reported a prevalence of 2.60% [8]. In 2012 Ortega et al. published a retrospective case series on incidental findings on CT-scans of children with mild head trauma at a single university medical center. They reported a prevalence of ACs of 1.30% ($n = 524$). Another year later, Al-Holou et al. [2] repeated their study on the prevalence of ACs with a study on adults who had undergone brain MRI at the university of Michigan health system between 1997 and 2009. Their series consisted of 47,417 patients, ACs were found in 661 patients (prevalence 1.40%). More recently, the results of the HUNT MRI study were published. It evaluated types and prevalence of all, incidental, and clinically relevant incidental intracranial findings, i.e., those referred to primary physician or clinical specialist, in a cohort between 50 and 66 years from the Nord-Trøndelag

Health study [9]. Among the 1006 participants 36 ACs were found (prevalence 3.60%). In the same year, Rabiei published another population-based study on the prevalence and symptoms of intracranial ACs [1]. The sample comprised a population-based cohort ($n = 1235$) aged older than 70 years. They described a prevalence of 2.30%. These results are summarized in Table 9.1.

Raw mean prevalence is 1.10% [1.07%−1.19%]. The fixed effects model calculates a prevalence of 1.40% [1.32%−1.48%]; the random effects model a prevalence of 1.20% [0.80%−1.99%]. The raw mean prevalence treats each of the 10 studies equally, whereas the effect models use weighted averages of the individual study effect, the weights being inversely proportional to the within study variances. The fixed effects model assumes to estimate a true single effect size (prevalence), the random effects model assumes the prevalence of each study to have been sampled from a distribution of prevalences. In summary, the random

TABLE 9.1 Prevalence of Arachnoid Cysts

Study	Cases	Sample Size	Proportion	95%-CI	%W (fixed)	%W (random)
[3]	86	27,187	0.0032	[0.0025; 0.0039]	6.7	10.8
[4]	43	2389	0.0180	[0.0131; 0.0242]	3.3	10.6
[5]	22	2000	0.0110	[0.0069; 0.0166]	1.7	10.2
[6]	2	478	0.0042	[0.0005; 0.0150]	0.2	5.7
[7]	99	19,559	0.0051	[0.0041; 0.0062]	7.7	10.9
[8]	309	11,738	0.0263	[0.0235; 0.0294]	23.6	11.0
[10]	7	524	0.0134	[0.0054; 0.0273]	0.5	8.7
[2]	661	48,417	0.0137	[0.0126; 0.0147]	51.2	11.0
[9]	36	1006	0.0358	[0.0252; 0.0492]	2.7	10.5
[1]	29	1235	0.0235	[0.0158; 0.0336]	2.2	10.4

95%-CI, 95% confidence interval; %W(fixed), percentage of the weight of the study, according to fixed effects or to a random effects (%W(random)) model.

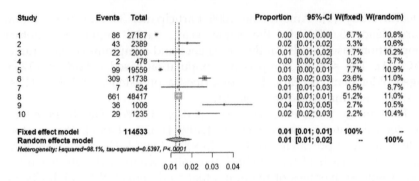

Study	Events	Total		Proportion	95%-CI	W(fixed)	W(random)
1	86	27187		0.00	[0.00; 0.00]	6.7%	10.8%
2	43	2389		0.02	[0.01; 0.02]	3.3%	10.6%
3	22	2000		0.01	[0.01; 0.02]	1.7%	10.2%
4	2	478		0.00	[0.00; 0.02]	0.2%	5.7%
5	99	19559		0.01	[0.00; 0.01]	7.7%	10.9%
6	309	11738		0.03	[0.02; 0.03]	23.6%	11.0%
7	7	524		0.01	[0.01; 0.03]	0.5%	8.7%
8	661	48417		0.01	[0.01; 0.01]	51.2%	11.0%
9	36	1006		0.04	[0.03; 0.05]	2.7%	10.5%
10	29	1235		0.02	[0.02; 0.03]	2.2%	10.4%
Fixed effect model		114533		0.01	[0.01; 0.01]	100%	--
Random effects model				0.01	[0.01; 0.02]	--	100%

Heterogeneity: I-squared=98.1%, tau-squared=0.5397, P<.0001

0.01 0.02 0.03 0.04

FIGURE 9.1   Forest plot showing the prevalence estimates from various studies.

TABLE 9.2   Intracranial Distribution of Arachnoid Cysts

Study	n	Male	Female	Temporal			Frontal	Parieto-occipital	Post. fossa	Other
				R	L					
[3]	86			28			15	25	11	7
[11]	55	38	17	43	15	28	11	1	0	0
[4]	43	43		31	7	19	5		5	3
[12]	156	95	61	113	33	77	24		13	6
[2]	309			145	49	96	18		118	28
[13]	299	183	116	204	54	137	42		36	23
[14]	75	54	21	48				5	13	9
[2]	696	356	305	237	71	166	4	98	353	4
[1]	29	6	25	16	5	11	2		13	

R, right; L, left.

effects models' prevalence of 1.20% seems to give the most realistic estimate, providing a more conservative 95% confidence interval that covers the confidence intervals of the former calculations.

A forest plot with the corresponding information is given in Fig. 9.1.

There is strong evidence for heterogeneity ($Q = 468$) between the 10 studies, reflecting their different origins, e.g., in the population-based studies (Rotterdam, Kumar, HUNT, Rabiei) there is a raw mean prevalence of $89/4719 = 1.89\%$, which is significantly larger than the raw mean prevalence of the hospital-based studies ($1205/109{,}814 = 1.10\%$).

The prevalence of ACs does not change significantly with advancing age in adulthood [2,3], see Chapter 11, Growth and Disappearance of Arachnoid Cysts.

Concerning the intracranial distribution of the ACs, with the exception of the study of Rabiei et al. and of Weber and Knopf, there are only data from hospital-based patient studies available, possibly reflecting a selection bias. The categorization differs between the studies, leaving a substantial proportion of "other" locations (Table 9.2).

In this collection, the proportion of men is higher (59%) and cysts in the middle cranial fossa count for about 50% of all ACs. The next most frequent location is the posterior fossa with about one-third of all cysts. In the frontal and in the parietotemporal regions are in each case about 7%, and the rest (5%) elsewhere. Temporal cysts are in 70% left-sided. There is a location-related sidedness for ACs, independent of patient sex.

For the calculations, the software R, version 3.2.3 for Mac OS X, and the package "meta," version 4.4-1, were used.

References

[1] Rabiei K, Jaraj D, Marlow T, Jensen C, Skoog I, Carsten Wikkelsø C. Prevalence and symptoms of intracranial arachnoid cysts: a population-based study. J Neurol 2016;263:689−94.

[2] Al-Holou WN, Terman S, Kilburg C, Garton HJL, Muraszko KM, Maher CO. Prevalence and natural history of arachnoid cysts in adults. J Neurosurg 2013;118:222−31.

[3] Becker T, Wagner M, Hofmann E, Warmuth-Metz M, Nadjmi M. Do arachnoid cysts grow? Neuroradiology 1991;33:341−5.

[4] Weber F, Knopf H. Incidental findings in magnetic resonance imaging of the brains of healthy young men. J Neurol Sci 2006;240(1−2):81−4.

[5] Vernooij MW, Ikram MA, Tanghe HL, Vincent AJPE, Hofman A, Krestin GP, et al. Incidental findings on brain MRI in the general population. N Engl J Med 2007;357:1821−8.

[6] Kumar R, Sachdev PS, Price JL, Rosenman S, Christensen H. Incidental brain MRI abnormalities in 60- to 64-year-old community-dwelling individuals: data from the Personalit y and Total Health Through Life study. Acta Neuropsychiatrica 2008;20: 87−90.

[7] Morris Z, Whiteley W, Longstreth N, Weber WT, Yi-Chung Lee F, Tsushima Y, et al. Incidental findings on brain magnetic resonance imaging: systematic review and meta-analysis. BMJ 2009;339:b3016. Available from: http://dx.doi.org/10.1136/bmj. b3016.

[8] Al-Holou WN, Yew YA, Boomsaad ZE, Garton HJL, Muraszko KM, Maher CO. Prevalence and natural history of arachnoid cysts in children. J Neurosurg Pediatrics 2010;5:578−85.

[9] Håberg AK, Hammer TA, Kvistad KA, Rydland J, Müller TB, Eikenes L, et al. Incidental intracranial findings and their clinical impact; the HUNT MRI study in a general population of 1006 participants between 50−66 years. PLoS One 2016;11: e0151080.

[10] Ortega HW, Vander Velden H, Reid S. Incidental findings on computed tomography scans in children with mild headtrauma. Clin Pediatrics 2012;51:872−6.

[11] Raeder MB, Helland CA, Hugdahl K, Wester K. Arachnoid cysts cause cognitive deficits that improve after surgery. Neurology 2005;64:160−2.

[12] Helland CA, Wester K. A population-based study of intracranial arachnoid cysts-Clinical and radiological outcome following surgical cyst decompression in adults. J Neurol Neurosurg Psychiatry 2007;78:1129−35.
[13] Helland CA, Lund-Johansen M, Wester K. Location, sidedness, and sex distribution of intracranial arachnoid cysts in a population-based sample. J Neurosurg 2010;113: 934−9.
[14] Duz B, Kaya S, Daneyemez M, Gonul E. Surgical management strategies of intracranial arachnoid cysts: a single institution experience of 75 cases. Turkish Neurosurg 2012;22:591−8.

10

Classification and Location of Arachnoid Cysts

Christian A. Helland[1,2]

[1]University of Bergen, Bergen, Norway [2]Haukeland University Hospital, Bergen, Norway

ABBREVIATIONS

AC	arachnoid cyst
CT	computerized tomography
CTC	CT-Cisternogram
MRC	MR communication studies
MRI	magnetic resonance imaging
PC-MRI	phase-contrast cine magnetic resonance imaging

Arachnoid Cysts: Epidemiology, Biology, and Neuroimaging
DOI: http://dx.doi.org/10.1016/B978-0-12-809932-2.00010-7

INTRODUCTION

Arachnoid cysts (ACs) are found in relation to arachnoid membranes along the entire neuraxis. Based on 208 reported cases in the literature, Rengachary and Wantanabe found the following distribution in their pioneer study from 1981: Sylvian fissure 103 (49%), cerebellopontine angle 22 (11%), supracollicular area 21 (10%), vermian area 19 (9%), sellar and suprasellar area 18 (9%), interhemispheric fissure 10 (5%), cerebral convexity 9 (4%), and clival area 6 (3%) [1].

The above figures were based on literature published from 1831 through 1980, most diagnosed postmortem and in the pre-CT era. It is thus conceivable that patients with severe symptoms were overrepresented in this study, which might have interfered with the reported distribution of both intracranial location and sidedness of AC.

The increasingly widespread use of computerized imaging (computed tomography (CT) and magnetic resonance imaging (MRI)) has undoubtedly lowered the threshold for radiological investigations of patients with headache, which is the dominating symptom in patients with intracranial AC. As a consequence, the diagnosis of an AC is now made more often than before. In a population-based patient material from our institution, the intracranial distribution among 299 patients with 305 cysts (six patients with bitemporal cysts) was as follows: the vast majority—198 patients (66.2%)—had cysts located in the middle cranial fossa (included the six patients with bitemporal cysts), 42 (14%) had frontal cysts, 36 (12%) had cysts in the posterior fossa, and 23 (7.7%) had cysts located in various other places within the neurocranium [2]. These numbers correspond well with other studies on intracranial distribution from the CT era [3].

In the same population, cysts in the middle fossa demonstrated a significant preponderance for the left side in both genders. A similar significant sidedness was found for cysts located in the cerebellopontine angle, although on the right side [2].

After its introduction, CT quickly became the standard neuroimaging technique for detection and characterization of AC [3–10]. On CT, the cyst is usually seen as a low-density lesion, with attenuation values similar to those of cerebrospinal fluid (CSF). It has well-defined margins, and the cyst wall does not enhance after intravenous contrast injection.

Intrathecal contrast infusion may add valuable information. Preoperatively, it is possible to verify that an intracranial fluid compartment truly is a cyst, and postoperatively it may be clarified if a previous cyst fenestration remains open [7,8,10–12] (see also Chapter 14, Radiological Workup, CT, MRI).

The advent of MRI has improved the diagnostics of intracranial ACs, especially for posterior fossa cysts, and it is now the standard neuroimaging technique for detection and characterization of AC [4,13−34]. MRI signals are similar to CSF in T1- and T2-weighted imaging with no enhancement on gadolinium.

MRI allows functional imaging of the neighboring cerebral tissue, and thereby direct assessment of any functional impairment caused by the AC, pre- and postoperatively [21,22,25]. Other sequences, such as flow-sensitive cine MRI techniques, have added valuable tools in the practical/clinical classification of cysts into so-called communicating and noncommunicating [24,35].

Positron emission tomography (PET) and single-photon emission computed tomography (SPECT) are other neuroimaging modalities that have brought valuable insight into the pathophysiology of AC, as they have been shown to reveal cyst induced hypo-metabolism and hypo-perfusion in neighboring cerebral tissue [16,36−44], see Chapter 16, SPECT Studies in Patients With Arachnoid Cysts. However, these techniques have not been used as a clinical routine.

CLASSIFICATION OF MIDDLE FOSSA TEMPORAL CYSTS—GALASSI CLASSIFICATION

Based on CT scan and (metrizamide) CT-cisternography (CTC), Galassi et al. provided a useful classification of middle fossa ACs based on their size, the segment of the Sylvian fissure involved, evidence of a mass effect, and the presence or absence of what they referred to as communication with the subarachnoid space (Fig. 10.1A−C) [10].

In the original publication by Galassi et al., seven patients were investigated with metrizamide CTC. Serial images were obtained at 1, 3, 6, 12, and 24 hours.

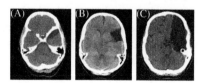

FIGURE 10.1 Illustrations of Galassi type I-III. (A) Type I is small, biconvex, and located at the anterior temporal pole. No radiological mass effect. (B) Type II involves the proximal and intermediate segments of the Sylvian fissure. The completely open insula gives a rectangular shape. (C) Type III involves the entire Sylvian fissure. It has often a marked radiological mass effect.

In this classification, a type I cyst is described as "the mildest form of ACs. The lesion is small, spindle-shaped, and limited to the anterior aspect of the temporal fossa. The temporal pole is compressed posteriorly. An appreciable mass effect is always lacking on CT scans, with no displacement or distortion of the ventricles and midline structures. Cranial deformities and angiographic abnormalities are absent or negligible."

On communication studies these cysts (two cases) were massively filled with metrizamide at the first CT examination, 1 hour after the intrathecal injection, as were the basal cisterns. Maximum enhancement occurred after 3 hours. At 12 hours the lesion seemed almost completely cleared of the contrast medium.

The larger cyst type was described in the following way: "Type II is the classic type as described by Banna. The lesion is medium-sized and its shape is roughly triangular or quadrangular, at least on one slice on the CT scan, with a straight inner margin. It occupies the anterior and middle part of the temporal fossa and extends superiorly along the sylvian fissure, which is therefore widely open with the insula exposed. The temporal lobe is clearly foreshortened. A mass effect, though not particularly severe, was seen in more than half of the patients. Cranial deformities on plain radiograms and angiographic abnormalities were constantly detectable, but sometimes of a moderate degree."

On communication studies (two cases), metrizamide penetration was absent or negligible on the 1-hour CT-cisternograms; it became quite evident at 3 hours, and reached a maximum at 6 hours.

Drainage of contrast from the lesion was delayed compared with type I cysts and the subarachnoid space. At the 12-hour examination the metrizamide staining of the cyst was still clearly detectable; furthermore, at 24 hours the intracystic density, although markedly decreased, was still higher than the standard values for CSF.

This is how they described the largest cyst type: "Type III cyst is the most severe form. The cyst is huge and appears oval or round. It occupies the temporal fossa almost entirely and extends over a wide area of the cerebral hemispheres, splitting the opercula of the sylvian fissure. The temporal lobe is severely atrophic and both the frontal and parietal lobes are extensively compressed, so that a large part of the one side of the cranial cavity may be occupied. A striking mass effect is the rule. The ventricles and midline structures are noticeably and sometimes tremendously distorted and pushed contralaterally. Cranial deformities and angiographic pathological changes are constantly found and very pronounced."

On communication studies these cysts (three cases) had a different pattern than type I and II cysts. No clear contrast filling was observed in two out of three cases at early or late cisternograms. In the third case, an appreciable staining of the lesion occurred, but with lower attenuation values and noticeable delay compared with types I and II. The contrast concentration reached its peak late, at 24 hours.

Based on these communication studies, Galassi et al. assumed the presence of communication in type I and II cysts, whereas type III lesions did not communicate with the rest of the subarachnoid space.

How to interpret the Galassi observations—is it certain that they show direct communication?

Whether the contrast filling of the cyst in the hours after intrathecal injection, as observed by Galassi et al., represents a true and direct communication between the cyst and the subarachnoid space is questionable. A significant confounder in this respect is the time that elapsed from intrathecal administration of contrast to the first CT scanning (1 hour) [10]. With this time span, it is conceivable, perhaps even probable, that the cyst was filled by *diffusion* over the thin cyst membrane of the water-soluble metrizamide rather than by a direct communication. A diffusion mechanism could explain why the contrast density is more pronounced in a small volume cyst (type I) than in a large one (type III). Furthermore, this investigation was performed in the early CT era (from 1970 to 1981), with single-slice scanners. The partial volume effect in a single-slice scanner with thick slices will have the same apparent effect as diffusion in a communication study; namely that smaller cysts might appear (partly) contrast-filled, while larger cysts do not.

OTHER LOCATIONS

A more recent study of intracranial ACs using Omnipaque CTC with the same temporal resolution as Galassi (1, 3, 6, 12, and 24 hours) to evaluate communication, but with a later (48 hours) scan to evaluate clearance time suggested a clinical classification of cysts (complete, incomplete, and noncommunicating cysts), also in other locations than the temporal fossa [12], such as the posterior fossa (Fig. 10.2). However, the same confounder regarding communication or not is the time elapsed from intrathecal administration of contrast to the first CT scanning (1 hour).

By adding intrathecal gadolinium (gadopentetate dimeglumine) MR cisternography (MRC) can provide the same information as CTC. In their study, Tali et al. performed the MR scan immediately after the administration of gadolinum intrathecally, so their classification of AC as communicating or noncommunicating cysts are not confounded by the possible time dependent diffusion of contrast [27].

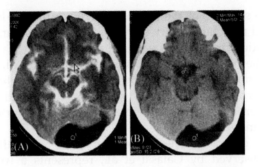

FIGURE 10.2 Noncommunicating cyst located in cisterna magna. (A) CTC image showing no filling of the cyst 3 h after intrathecal injection. (B) CTC image showing a slight contrast filling of the cyst 24 h after intrathecal injection. *Reprinted from Wang X, Chen JX, You C, Jiang S. CT cisternography in intracranial symptomatic arachnoid cysts: classification and treatment. J Neurol Sci. 2012;318(1−2):125−130 with permission from Elsevier.*

Classification of temporal cysts in communicating/noncommunicating cysts has also been described using phase-contrast cine magnetic resonance imaging (PC-MRI) [45,46].

Overall, it is our firm belief that communication studies (both CTC and MRC) must be performed with as little delay as possible between intrathecal contrast injection and scanning to avoid false classification of a cyst as communicating.

Both techniques (CTC/PC-MRI/MRC) also provide a useful tool in evaluating the stoma between the cyst and its adjacent cistern postoperatively in cases where there is doubt if the fenestration is still open (see also Chapter 14, Radiological Workup, CT, MRI).

Suprasellar Cysts

Suprasellar ACs (SACs) display some distinct features, such as development later in embryological development, de novo formation, and an overrepresentation in cases with documented growth [47] (see also Chapter 11, Growth and Disappearance of Arachnoid Cysts). These features separate them from ACs with other intracranial locations to such a degree that SAC perhaps should be regarded as a separate entity, with a mechanism of development that differs from other intracranial AC, namely through defects or diverticula of the membrane of Liliequist and that upward herniation of the apical leaflet caused by CSF pulsations in the prepontine cistern can result in a communicating cyst with a one-way valve at the point where the basilar artery passes through the basal leaflet [48−51]. A separate classification of SAC has been proposed to guide decision-making in the treatment of SAC [52].

References

[1] Rengachary SS, Watanabe I. Ultrastructure and pathogenesis of intracranial arachnoid cysts. J Neuropathol Exp Neurol 1981;40(1):61−83.

[2] Helland CA, Lund-Johansen M, Wester K. Location, sidedness, and sex distribution of intracranial arachnoid cysts in a population-based sample. J Neurosurg 2010;113 (5):934−9.

[3] Wester K. Gender distribution and sidedness of middle fossa arachnoid cysts: a review of cases diagnosed with computed imaging. Neurosurgery 1992;31(5):940−4.

[4] Go KG. The diagnosis and treatment of intracranial arachnoid cysts. Neurosurg Quart 1995;5(3):187−204.

[5] Galassi E, Gaist G, Giuliani G, Pozzati E. Arachnoid cysts of the middle cranial fossa: experience with 77 cases treated surgically. Acta Neurochir Suppl (Wien) 1988;42:201−4.

[6] Garcia-Bach M, Isamat F, Vila F. Intracranial arachnoid cysts in adults. Acta Neurochir Suppl (Wien) 1988;42:205−9.

[7] Hoffman HJ, Hendrick EB, Humphreys RP, Armstrong EA. Investigation and management of suprasellar arachnoid cysts. J Neurosurg 1982/11;57(5):597−602.

[8] Locatelli D, Bonfanti N, Sfogliarini R, Gajno TM, Pezzotta S. Arachnoid cysts: diagnosis and treatment. Childs Nerv Syst 1987;3(2):121−4.

[9] Eskandary H, Sabba M, Khajehpour F, Eskandari M. Incidental findings in brain computed tomography scans of 3000 head trauma patients. Surg Neurol 2005;63 (6):550−3.

[10] Galassi E, Tognetti F, Gaist G, Fagioli L, Frank F, Frank G. CT scan and metrizamide CT cisternography in arachnoid cysts of the middle cranial fossa: classification and pathophysiological aspects. Surg Neurol 1982;17(5):363−9.

[11] Hayashi T, Anegawa S, Honda E, Kuramoto S, Mori K, Murata T, et al. Clinical analysis of arachnoid cysts in the middle fossa. Neurochirurgia (Stuttg) 1979/11;22 (6):201−10.

[12] Wang X, Chen JX, You C, Jiang S. CT cisternography in intracranial symptomatic arachnoid cysts: classification and treatment. J Neurol Sci 2012;318(1−2):125−30.

[13] Patel TR, Bannister CM, Thorne J. A study of prenatal ultrasound and postnatal magnetic imaging in the diagnosis of central nervous system abnormalities. Eur J Pediatr Surg 2003/12;13(Suppl 1):S18−22.

[14] Iqbal J, Kanaan I, Al HM. Non-neoplastic cystic lesions of the sellar region presentation, diagnosis and management of eight cases and review of the literature. Acta Neurochir (Wien) 1999;141(4):389−97.

[15] Jallo GI, Woo HH, Meshki C, Epstein FJ, Wisoff JH. Arachnoid cysts of the cerebellopontine angle: diagnosis and surgery. Neurosurgery 1997;40(1):31−7.

[16] Zaatreh MM, Bates ER, Hooper SR, Palmer G, Elmenshawi EE, Courvoisie HE, et al. Morphometric and neuropsychologic studies in children with arachnoid cysts. Pediatr Neurol 2002;26(2):134−8.

[17] Gandy SE, Heier LA. Clinical and magnetic resonance features of primary intracranial arachnoid cysts. Ann Neurol 1987;21(4):342−8.

[18] von Wild K, Gullotta F. Arachnoid cyst of the middle cranial fossa--aplasia of temporal lobe? Childs NervSyst 1987;3(4):232−4.

[19] Ibarra R, Kesava PP. Role of MR imaging in the diagnosis of complicated arachnoid cyst. Pediatr Radiol 2000/5;30(5):329−31.

[20] Vatsal DK, Husain M, Husain N, Chawla S, Roy R, Gupta RK. Cerebellar hemangioblastoma simulating arachnoid cyst on imaging and surgery. Neurosurg Rev 2002;25 (1−2):107−9.

[21] Alkadhi H, Crelier GR, Imhof HG, Kollias SS. Somatomotor functional MRI in a large congenital arachnoid cyst. Neuroradiology 2003;45(3):153−6.

[22] Caruso R, Colonnese C. Somatomotor functional MRI in a hypertensive arachnoid cyst. Acta Neurochir (Wien) 2006;148(7):801−3.

[23] Hakyemez B, Yildiz H, Ergin N, Uysal S, Parlak M. Flair and diffusion weighted MR imaging in differentiating epidermoid cysts from arachnoid cysts. Tani Girisim Radyol 2003;9(4):418−26.

[24] Hoffmann KT, Hosten N, Meyer BU, Roricht S, Sprung C, Oellinger J, et al. CSF flow studies of intracranial cysts and cyst-like lesions achieved using reversed fast imaging with steady-state precession MR sequences. AJNR Am J Neuroradiol 2000;21 (3):493−502.

[25] Hund-Georgiadis M, Yves Von CD, Kruggel F, Preul C. Do quiescent arachnoid cysts alter CNS functional organization?: a fMRI and morphometric study. Neurology 2002;59(12):1935−9.

[26] Pierre-Kahn A, Sonigo P. Malformative intracranial cysts: diagnosis and outcome. Childs Nerv Syst 2003;19(7-8):477−83.

[27] Tali ET, Ercan N, Kaymaz M, Pasaoglu A, Jinkins JR. Intrathecal gadolinium (gadopentetate dimeglumine)-enhanced MR cisternography used to determine potential communication between the cerebrospinal fluid pathways and intracranial arachnoid cysts. Neuroradiology 2004;46(9):744−54.

[28] Kusaka Y, Luedemann W, Oi S, Shwardfegar R, Samii M. Fetal arachnoid cyst of the quadrigeminal cistern in MRI and ultrasound. Childs Nerv Syst 2005;21(12):1065−6.

[29] Tsuruda JS, Chew WM, Moseley ME, Norman D. Diffusion-weighted MR imaging of the brain: value of differentiating between extraaxial cysts and epidermoid tumors. AJR Am J Roentgenol 1990/11;155(5):1059−65.

[30] Kuzma BB, Goodman JM. Epidermoid or arachnoid cyst? Surg Neurol 1997/4;47 (4):395−6.

[31] Tien RD, MacFall J, Heinz R. Evaluation of complex cystic masses of the brain: value of steady-state free-precession MR imaging. AJR Am J Roentgenol 1992/11;159 (5):1049−55.

[32] Yildiz H, Yazici Z, Hakyemez B, Erdogan C, Parlak M. Evaluation of CSF flow patterns of posterior fossa cystic malformations using CSF flow MR imaging. Neuroradiology 2006/9;48(9):595−605.

[33] Tan EC, Takagi T, Karasawa K. Posterior fossa cystic lesions--magnetic resonance imaging manifestations. Brain Dev 1995;17(6):418−24.

[34] Thorat JD, Sitoh YY, Chin CH, Ng I. Diffusion tensor imaging in a symptomatic patient with an intra-axial arachnoid cyst. Br J Neurosurg 2006/4;20(2):94−6.

[35] Eguchi T, Taoka T, Nikaido Y, Shiomi K, Fujimoto T, Otsuka H, et al. Cine-magnetic resonance imaging evaluation of communication between middle cranial fossa arachnoid cysts and cisterns. Neurol Med Chir (Tokyo) 1996;36(6):353−7.

[36] Martinez-Lage JF, Ruiz-Macia D, Valenti JA, Poza M. Development of a middle fossa arachnoid cyst. A theory on its pathogenesis. Childs Nerv Syst 1999;15(2-3):94−7.

[37] De Volder AG, Michel C, Thauvoy C, Willems G, Ferriere G. Brain glucose utilisation in acquired childhood aphasia associated with a sylvian arachnoid cyst: recovery after shunting as demonstrated by PET. J Neurol Neurosurg Psychiatry 1994;57 (3):296−300.

[38] Horiguchi T, Takeshita K. Cognitive function and language of a child with an arachnoid cyst in the left frontal fossa. World J BiolPsychiatry 2000;1(3):159−63.

[39] Martinez-Lage JF, Valenti JA, Piqueras C, Ruiz-Espejo AM, Roman F, NdlR JA. Functional assessment of intracranial arachnoid cysts with TC99 m-HMPAO SPECT: a preliminary report. Childs Nerv Syst 2006;22(9):1091−7.

III. PREVALENCE AND NATURAL HISTORY OF ARACHNOID CYSTS

[40] Sgouros S, Chapman S. Congenital middle fossa arachnoid cysts may cause global brain ischaemia: a study with 99Tc-hexamethylpropyleneamineoxime single photon emission computerised tomography scans. Pediatr Neurosurg 2001;35(4):188−94.

[41] Sato H, Sato N, Katayama S, Tamaki N, Matsumoto S. Effective shunt-independent treatment for primary middle fossa arachnoid cyst. Childs Nerv Syst 1991;7 (7):375−81.

[42] Holman BL, Zimmerman RE, Johnson KA, Carvalho PA, Schwartz RB, Loeffler JS, et al. Computer-assisted superimposition of magnetic resonance and high-resolution technetium-99m-HMPAO and thallium-201 SPECT images of the brain. J Nucl Med 1991/8;32(8):1478−84.

[43] Stowe LA, Go KG, Pruim J, den DW, Meiners LC, Paans AM. Language localization in cases of left temporal lobe arachnoid cyst: evidence against interhemispheric reorganization. Brain Lang 2000;75(3):347−58.

[44] Tsurushima H, Harakuni T, Saito A, Tominaga D, Hyodo A, Yoshii Y. Symptomatic arachnoid cyst of the left frontal convexity presenting with memory disturbance-- case report. Neurol (Tokyo) 2000;40(6):339−41.

[45] Li L, Zhang Y, Li Y, Zhai X, Zhou Y, Liang P. The clinical classification and treatment of middle cranial fossa arachnoid cysts in children. Clin Neurol Neurosurg 2013;115 (4):411−18.

[46] Yildiz H, Erdogan C, Yalcin R, Yazici Z, Hakyemez B, Parlak M, et al. Evaluation of communication between intracranial arachnoid cysts and cisterns with phase-contrast cine MR imaging. AJNR Am J Neuroradiol 2005;26(1):145−51.

[47] Invergo D, Tomita T. De novo suprasellar arachnoid cyst: case report and review of the literature. Pediatr Neurosurg 2012;48(3):199−203.

[48] Fox JL, Al-Mefty O. Suprasellar arachnoid cysts: an extension of the membrane of Liliequist. Neurosurgery 1980;7(6):615−18.

[49] Miyajima M, Arai H, Okuda O, Hishii M, Nakanishi H, Sato K. Possible origin of suprasellar arachnoid cysts: neuroimaging and neurosurgical observations in nine cases. J Neurosurg 2000;93(1):62−7.

[50] Santamarta D, Aguas J, Ferrer E. The natural history of arachnoid cysts: endoscopic and cine-mode MRI evidence of a slit-valve mechanism. Minim Invasive Neurosurg 1995;38(4):133−7.

[51] Schroeder HW, Gaab MR. Endoscopic observation of a slit-valve mechanism in a suprasellar prepontine arachnoid cyst: case report. Neurosurgery 1997;40(1):198−200.

[52] Andre A, Zerah M, Roujeau T, Brunelle F, Blauwblomme T, Puget S, et al. Suprasellar arachnoid cysts: toward a new simple classification based on prognosis and treatment modality. Neurosurgery 2016;78(3):370−9 discussion 9−80.

11

Growth and Disappearance of Arachnoid Cysts

Knut Wester[1,2]

[1]University of Bergen, Bergen, Norway [2]Haukeland University Hospital, Bergen, Norway

OUTLINE

ABBREVIATIONS

AC arachnoid cyst
BEH benign external hydrocephalus
BESS benign enlargement of the subarachnoid spaces

Arachnoid Cysts: Epidemiology, Biology, and Neuroimaging
DOI: http://dx.doi.org/10.1016/B978-0-12-809932-2.00011-9

CNS   central nervous system
CT   computerized tomography
MRI magnetic resonance imaging

Judged by the existing literature, growth of an arachnoid cyst after early childhood is extremely rare. Many colleagues advocate a strategy of repeated neuroimaging procedures to see if the cyst grows. As cyst growth has been demonstrated in only five adults worldwide, this strategy seems to lack any rationality. The probability of ever seeing an AC grow appears close to zero, except for in children below 3 years-of-age.

RECOMMENDATIONS—LEVEL OF EVIDENCE

Level I

There is no Level I evidence available for topics covered in this chapter.

Level II

De novo postnatal AC development has only been demonstrated in young children, mostly infants. Cyst enlargement of an already existing AC in children is associated with very young age and takes place mainly in infancy.

Level III

Growth of an AC in adults is very rare. Disappearance of an AC is the most commonly reported spontaneous change in cyst size and may occur both in children and adults.

Arachnoid cysts (ACs) are usually regarded as congenital and stable cysts that do not change much in size, unless they have provoked subdural or intracystic bleeding, which they are known to do, although quite rarely [1] (see also Chapter 12, Arachnoid Cysts and Subdural and Intracystic Hematomas). However, occasional reports have been published that indicate de novo (postnatal) AC development, growth of existing ACs, or spontaneous disappearance of an AC, see Table 11.1 for a summary.

Judged by the number of publications, cyst disappearance appears to be more common than the postnatal growth, as will be demonstrated in the following. All such events appear, however, to occur quite

TABLE 11.1   Table showing a summary of the cases and publications described in this chapter. Numbers in [ ] refer to the cited publications

	Age		
	0–1 year	1– <16 years	>16 years
De novo-case stories [47–54]	3	5	–
De novo-prospective study [55]	18 pediatric patients—mean 19.5 months		
Postnatal growth-case stories [19,53,57–60]	3	1	5
Postnatal growth—prospective study [3]	14	3 (1–3 years)	–
Spontaneous disappearance—case stories [9–34]	4	19	6

infrequently; it is therefore only to be expected that most of these reports are single case stories or small case series.

To my knowledge, only two patient cohort studies have tried to investigate whether ACs grow [2,3]. The main finding in the oldest study [2] is that there seems to be a statistically significant correlation between patient age and volume for cysts larger than the volumetric mean, but not so for cysts smaller than the mean. This finding may indicate that a subgroup of ACs may grow with age, but cannot be regarded as evidence for that. Moreover, this finding has not been confirmed in other studies. A small subgroup of 11 nonoperated patients in the same study was followed with sequential CT scanning and cyst volume measurements. According to the authors' judgment, three of these cysts increased in size, six remained unchanged on the follow-up scans, and a volume reduction was seen in the last two. The exact follow-up time is however not given; from their Fig. 11.2 it appears to be in the magnitude of months to a few years at the most, and the changes in volume seem rather moderate.

In a more recent study [3], 86 children younger than 5 years-of-age with an AC were followed with neuroimaging. Changes of the cysts' size were determined and plotted on individual graphs. The children were divided into four different age groups (0–0.5 year, 0.5–1 year, 1–3 years, and 3–5 years). These authors found that cyst enlargement over time took place in 17 children (19.8%); the majority (14) were younger than 12 months. Cyst enlargement was never seen above the age of 3. In six patients, the cyst enlargement ceased, and spontaneous volume reduction was observed in three patients. Age at diagnosis of the AC was the only significant factor associated with cyst enlargement.

This finding of Lee et al.—that changes in cyst size mainly occur in the youngest individuals—receives support from the many case stories referred to in the sections below. This applies above all to de novo cysts that with certainty have developed after birth; this phenomenon has only been reported in 26 young children, mostly infants, and never in adults. Further growth of an already diagnosed cyst may however occur in older individuals as well; five of the nine patients reported in these case stories were adults (age range 23—81 years). Spontaneous cyst disappearance or resolution has also been described in adults, however, most often in children.

In addition, Arunkumar et al. have also published one adult patient with considerable spontaneous volume fluctuations in a posterior fossa AC [4].

More detailed information on these three events (spontaneous disappearance, de novo development, and further growth of an AC) are given below.

SPONTANEOUS DISAPPEARANCE OR REDUCTION OF CYSTS

A literature search was performed, using these search words: "arachnoid cyst AND spontaneous* disappear* OR spontaneous* reduc* OR spontaneous* resol*." Cases with a CNS infection preceding the disappearance [5] or where the cyst disappeared after any, however minimal, intracranial surgical procedure, were not included [6]. Excluded was also one report of a cyst that only was *presumed* to be an AC and that was diagnosed and disappeared in utero before an exact diagnosis could be made [7]. In addition, a report that describes the spontaneous disappearance of a minute cystic lesion in the right Meckel's cave was not included [8]. Twenty-seven reports from the period 1985—2016 describing a total of 28 patients with a mean age of 14 years (range 0—80 years) were included in the survey [9—35]. Most of these patients were children; 23 patients were 16 years or younger, four of them infants. Only six patients were adults (Fig. 11.1).

The majority of the cysts (18) that disappeared were located in the middle fossa (left/right ratio: 10/8), 16 males and two females. Five cysts had a prepontine/suprasellar location, three were overlying the frontal cortex, and two were found in the posterior fossa. There was a marked preponderance of male patients in the survey, 21 males versus 6 females, mainly because of the large number of males in the middle fossa cyst group. Gender was not given for one infant. The distribution of cyst locations does not seem to deviate much from the distribution one can find in large, population-based patient cohorts [36]. In addition to the cysts included in the survey above, a suprasellar cyst has been

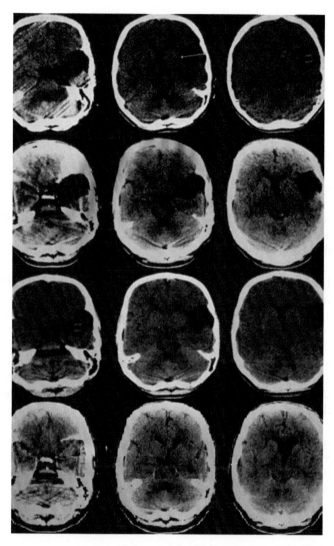

FIGURE 11.1   CT scan of an 11-year-old boy with epilepsy and moderate behavioral disorder (upper row). A left temporal AC was diagnosed, but not operated; the cyst remained stable at 13 and 18 years of age (2 middle rows). After a moderate and transitory increase in seizure activity at the age of 21, a control CT was performed to rule out an unexpected event. Rather surprisingly, the cyst had then disappeared completely without any known trauma. The patient is described in more detail in Wester et al. [33]. *Reprinted from Wester K, et al. Spontaneous disappearance of an arachnoid cyst in the middle intracranial fossa. Neurology 1991;41(9):1524−1526 with permission of Wolters Kluwer©.*

published that first disappeared spontaneously and reappeared larger than before 1 month later [37].

POSTNATAL DEVELOPMENT OF DE NOVO ACs AND GROWTH OF AN ESTABLISHED AC

Whether an AC is congenital (i.e., present at birth) or it develops postnatally, is in most cases impossible to know. A prerequisite for detecting postnatal development of a new AC is that the child for some reason already has undergone an initial neuroimaging procedure that failed to reveal a cyst and that a subsequent radiological procedure is performed, precipitated by symptoms that most likely are different from those causing the first investigation. Such a series of unusual events must be very rare. Consequently, in most cases it is impossible to know whether a cyst developed before or after birth.

As will be apparent from below, existing literature indicates that ACs indeed can develop after birth; however, whether this is a true de novo development or just postnatal growth of a very small, preformed cyst that eluded detection by the first imaging, cannot be said with certainty.

Growth of an already existing AC is most probably caused by other mechanisms than those instrumental in development of a new cyst. Based on what we know about sidedness and gender preponderance of ACs [36,38,39] and from genetic studies [40,41], it is reasonable to assume that *formation* of an AC somehow is governed by some biological, most probably genetic, mechanisms. Growth of an already existing AC on the other hand is most probably simply caused by *filling* of the cyst with more fluid, either by a valve mechanism [42,43] or by active fluid transport or secretion across the cyst wall [44–46]. De novo development and growth of ACs will therefore be dealt with separately below.

Postnatal Development of De Novo ACs

A literature search for: "arachnoid cyst AND de novo OR spontaneous develop*" identified nine publications, eight of them being case reports [47–54]. Exactly *when* these cysts developed postnatally is not known, but the period during which it happened is reported. Three of these case reports describe suprasellar cysts that were not detected by neuroimaging at birth or at the ages of 6 weeks or 4 months, but that had developed on subsequent MRIs after 2 years, 2 years, and 4 years, respectively. In the remaining five cases, four middle fossa cysts developed during the time spans 2–5 months, 8–12 months, 13–22 months, and 2 days–7 years. One frontal cyst developed somewhere between birth and 4 years-of-age.

The relatively high number of suprasellar cysts in this small survey is surprising, as it does not correspond to the frequency one usually sees in larger patient cohorts [36,39]. This apparent overrepresentation may be incidental, but it may also be caused by a valve mechanism: the excess extracerebral fluid that one often sees in infants gets access to and fills a preformed space via a slit valve; such valves have been demonstrated only for suprasellar cysts, see below and Chapter 8, The "Valve Mechanism".

The by far most intriguing publication on postnatal development of new cysts, however, is that of Mattei et al. [55]. In this relatively large, prospective study comprising 44 children with "benign extracerebral fluid collections" (often referred to as BEH or BESS), the infants were followed up for 6 months from the initial diagnosis of the benign extra-cerebral fluid collection. Rather surprisingly, as many as 18 of these children (41%—16 boys, 2 girls) developed a new AC during the follow-up period, all located in the middle fossa, see Fig. 11.2. Nine of the cysts were located on the left side, four were found in the right middle fossa, and as many as five children had bitemporal cysts. The sidedness distri-bution is within what one can expect from previous population-based studies, but the relatively high proportion of bilateral cysts (27.8%) is indeed unexpected from previous studies [36,38,56].

The findings of Mattei et al. that there is a marked male preponder-ance in BEH children that develop a de novo AC in the temporal fossa is indeed interesting. We know from the literature that there also is a marked male preponderance in BEH children [57–61]. If it is true, as it

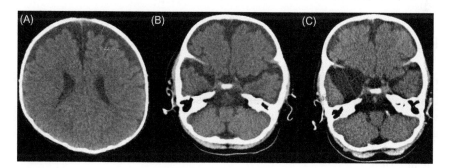

FIGURE 11.2 (A–B) Four-month-old child referred for evaluation of macrocephaly and mild developmental delay. Initial CT scan demonstrated excess extracerebral fluid col-lection and no evidence of AC. (C) control head CT scan 8 months later demonstrated development of a de novo right temporal AC. *Reprinted from Mattei TA. Pediatric arachnoid cysts and subdural hygromas in early infancy: challenging the direction of the causality paradigm. Neurosurgery E150 2014, January;74(1). With permission from Oxford Journals.*

appears from their study, that BEH predisposes only for development of *temporal* cysts, this coupling between BEH and temporal ACs may explain the marked male preponderance for cysts in this location [36,38].

The explanation offered by the authors appears to be that the association between such extracerebral fluid collections in infancy and the development of de novo ACs can be explained as the result of a "2-hit" process that starts with a meningeal maldevelopment causing an arachnoid dissection defect in the embryo. When this defect in early childhood is exposed to extracerebral fluid under pressure, as e.g., in benign external hydrocephalus (BEH), this fluid may enter the meningeal defect and blow up a preformed meningeal compartment— the second "hit." It then seems reasonable to assume that the filling and the expansion of the cyst is dependent on a unidirectional slit-valve mechanism.

The only problem with this model is that a slit-valve has been demonstrated only in suprasellar cysts [42,43] (see also Chapter 8, The "Valve Mechanism"), not with certainty in any other cyst locations.

Moreover, analyses of cyst fluid and genetic studies indicate that middle fossa cysts more likely are filled via fluid transport across the cyst wall rather than via a slit-valve [44,46]. Nevertheless, even if it is difficult to fully understand the underlying mechanisms, the association between BEH and AC as demonstrated by Mattei et al. must carry some important information. In this context it is noteworthy that also a de novo suprasellar cyst has been reported to be preceded by excess extracerebral fluid in infancy [51] and that one de novo temporal fossa AC developed between 13 and 22 months-of-age [52] in a baby that at the age of 13 months only had a moderate hydrocephalus.

Postnatal Growth of an Already Established AC

As already mentioned in the introduction to this chapter, Lee et al. [3] published a large prospective study comprising 86 children younger than 5 years-of-age that had been diagnosed with an AC. These children were followed-up with neuroimaging and it was found that further growth of the cyst took place in 17 children (19.8%); 14 of them were infants. A similar cyst enlargement was never seen in children above the age of 3.

For this section of the chapter, the literature was searched for: "arachnoid cyst AND grow* OR enlarge*." From this search, only six publications that describe a total of nine patients were identified [19,53,62—65]. As opposed to the systematic, prospective study by Lee et al. referred to above, these few case reports describe incidentally found cyst growth—also in adults (Fig. 11.3).

Five of the patients were 18 years-of-age or above when the cyst enlargement was discovered, the oldest being 81. Four of these nine growing cysts were located in the temporal fossa, four had a suprasellar location and one was located in the posterior fossa.

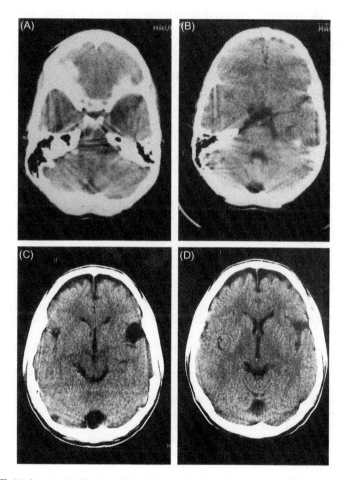

FIGURE 11.3 Axial CT scan of an 8-year-old boy showing a small arachnoid cyst in the left middle fossa (upper row). A control CT when the patient was 18 years old (lower row), showed that the cyst in the left middle fossa had grown considerably, now reaching well above the sphenoid wing. *Reproduced from Wester K, Moen G. Documented growth of a temporal arachnoid cyst. JNNP 2000; 69:699–700 with permission from BMJ Publishing Group Ltd.*

CONCLUSIVE REMARKS

ACs are among the most frequent intracranial expansions [66−69]. Bearing that in mind, changes in cyst volume, such as growth of already established cysts or spontaneous cyst disappearance, must be very rare, especially over the age of 18. Worldwide and until January 2017, a convincing and substantial growth of an already diagnosed AC has been reported in only five adult patients; similarly, cyst disappearance has been reported in only six adults (Table 11.1).

Instead of advising surgical treatment in adults, many neurologists and neurosurgeons prefer a conservative approach with repeated CT or MRI controls of the cyst. The assumed rationale for this strategy must be to postpone the decision to operate, and do so only if the cyst in fact grows. Taken into consideration how infrequently cyst enlargement has been reported, it seems highly unlikely that this policy will ever demonstrate growth or give any other sensible information useful for decision making.

My personal opinion is therefore that repeated neuroimaging controls in a patient with a symptomatic AC is a waste of time and resources. Besides, our experience from several independent studies is that the size of the cyst doesn't matter, neither for the strength of the complaints, nor for the results of surgery [70−72]. If a patient with an AC has strong and incapacitating symptoms, one has to make a decision on surgery there and then.

References

[1] Wester K, Helland CA. How often do chronic extra-cerebral haematomas occur in patients with intracranial arachnoid cysts? J Neurol Neurosurg Psychiatry 2008;79 (1):72−5.

[2] Becker T, et al. Do arachnoid cysts grow? A retrospective CT volumetric study. Neuroradiology 1991;33(4):341−5.

[3] Lee JY, et al. Enlarging arachnoid cyst: a false alarm for infants. Childs Nerv Syst 2012;28(8):1203−11.

[4] Arunkumar MJ, Haran RP, Chandy MJ. Spontaneous fluctuation in the size of a midline posterior fossa arachnoid cyst. Br J Neurosurg 1999;13(3):326−8.

[5] Yoshioka H, et al. Spontaneous disappearance of a middle cranial fossa arachnoid cyst after suppurative meningitis. Surg Neurol 1998;50(5):487−91.

[6] Moon KS, et al. Spontaneous disappearance of a suprasellar arachnoid cyst: case report and review of the literature. Childs Nerv Syst 2007;23(1):99−104.

[7] Elbers SE, Furness ME. Resolution of presumed arachnoid cyst in utero. Ultrasound Obstet Gynecol 1999;14(5):353−5.

[8] Jacob M, et al. Spontaneous resolution of a Meckel's cave arachnoid cyst causing sixth cranial nerve palsy. J Neuroophthalmol 2008;28(3):186−91.

[9] Beltramello A, Mazza C. Spontaneous disappearance of a large middle fossa arachnoid cyst. Surg Neurol 1985;24(2):181−3.

[10] Cokluk C, et al. Spontaneous disappearance of two asymptomatic arachnoid cysts in two different locations. Minim Inv Neurosurg 2003;46(2):110−12.

[11] Dodd RL, Barnes PD, Huhn SL. Spontaneous resolution of a prepontine arachnoid cyst-Case report and review of the literature. Pediat Neurosurg 2002;37(3):152−7.

[12] Gelabert-Gonzalez M, Serramito-Garcia R, Garcia-Allut A. Spontaneous resolution of an asymptomatic intracranial arachnoid cyst. Neurocirugia (Astur) 2008;19(4):361−4.

[13] Goksu E, Kazan S. Spontaneous shrinkage of a suprasellar arachnoid cyst diagnosed with prenatal sonography and fetal magnetic resonance imaging: case report and review of the literature. Turk Neurosurg 2015;25(4):670−3.

[14] Hanieh A, Simpson DA, North JB. Arachnoid cysts - a critical-review of 41 cases. Childs Nerv Syst 1988;4(2):92−6.

[15] Inoue T, et al. Spontaneous disappearance of a middle fossa arachnoid cyst associated with subdural hematoma. Surg Neurol 1987;28(6):447−50.

[16] Liu Z, Li J, Xu J. Teaching NeuroImages: spontaneous resolution of a giant intracranial arachnoid cyst. Neurology 2016;86(18):e199−200.

[17] Marlin E, Marlin A. Arachnoid cyst resolution. J Neurosurg Pediatr 2010;5(3):310−11.

[18] Matushita H, Cardeal DD, Monaco B. Spontaneous disappearance of cerebral convexity arachnoid cyst. Arq Neuropsiquiatr 2012;70(6):473−4.

[19] McDonald PJ, Rutka JT. Middle cranial fossa arachnoid cysts that come and go. Report of two cases and review of the literature. Pediatr Neurosurg 1997;26(1):48−52.

[20] Mokri B, Houser OW, Dinapoli RP. Spontaneous resolution of arachnoid cysts. J Neuroimaging 1994;4(3):165−8.

[21] Morbee L, et al. Spontaneous disappearance of arachnoid cyst after head trauma. Jbr-Btr 2015;99(1):107−8.

[22] Mori T, et al. Disappearance of arachnoid cysts after head injury. Neurosurgery 1995;36(5):938−41 discussion 941−2.

[23] Pandey P, et al. Spontaneous decompression of a posterior fossa arachnoid cyst: a case report. Pediatr Neurosurg 2001;35(3):162−3.

[24] Prokopienko M, Kunert P, Marchel A. Unusual volume reduction of Galassi grade III arachnoid cyst following head trauma. J Neurol Surg A Cent Eur Neurosurg 2013;74 (Suppl 1):e198−202.

[25] Przybylo HJ, et al. Spontaneous resolution of an asymptomatic arachnoid cyst. Pediatr Neurosurg 1997;26(6):312−14.

[26] Rakier A, Feinsod M. Gradual resolution of an arachnoid cyst after spontaneous rupture into the subdural space. Case report. J Neurosurg 1995;83(6):1085−6.

[27] Russo N, et al. Spontaneous reduction of intracranial arachnoid cysts: a complete review. Br J Neurosurg 2008;22(5):626−9.

[28] Shiono T, et al. A case of spontaneous disappearance of a middle fossa arachnoid cyst associated with subdural hematoma. Jpn J Clin Radiol 1993;38(8):921−3.

[29] Takagi K, Sasaki T, Basugi N. Spontaneous disappearance of cerebellopontine angle arachnoid cyst: report of a case. No Shinkei Geka 1987;15(3):295−9.

[30] Takizawa H, et al. Spontaneous disappearance of a middle fossa arachnoid cyst−a case report. No To Shinkei 1991;43(10):987−9.

[31] Thomas BP, Pearson MM, Wushensky CA. Active spontaneous decompression of a suprasellar-prepontine arachnoid cyst detected with routine magnetic resonance imaging. Case report. J Neurosurg Pediatr 2009;3(1):70−2.

[32] Weber R, et al. Spontaneous regression of a temporal arachnoid cyst. Childs Nerv Syst 1991;7(7):414−15.

[33] Wester K, et al. Spontaneous disappearance of an arachnoid cyst in the middle intracranial fossa. Neurology 1991;41(9):1524−6.

[34] Yamanouchi Y, Someda K, Oka N. Spontaneous disappearance of middle fossa arachnoid cyst after head injury. Childs Nerv Syst 1986;2(1):40−3.

[35] Yamauchi T, Saeki N, Yamaura A. Spontaneous disappearance of temporo-frontal arachnoid cyst in a child. Acta Neurochir (Wien) 1999;141(5):537−40.

[36] Helland CA, Lund-Johansen M, Wester K. Location, sidedness, and sex distribution of intracranial arachnoid cysts in a population-based sample. J Neurosurg 2010;113 (5):934−9.

[37] Bristol RE, et al. Arachnoid cysts: spontaneous resolution distinct from traumatic rupture. Case report. Neurosurg Focus 2007;22(2):E2.

[38] Wester K. Gender distribution and sidedness of middle fossa arachnoid cysts: a review of cases diagnosed with computed imaging. Neurosurgery 1992;31(5):940−4.

[39] Wester K. Peculiarities of intracranial arachnoid cysts: location, sidedness, and sex distribution in 126 consecutive patients. Neurosurgery 1999;45(4):775−9.

[40] Aarhus M, et al. Microarray-based gene expression profiling and DNA copy number variation analysis of temporal fossa arachnoid cysts. Cerebrospinal Fluid Res 2010;7:6.

[41] Helland CA, Wester K. Monozygotic twins with mirror image cysts: indication of a genetic mechanism in arachnoid cysts? Neurology 2007;69(1):110−11.

[42] Santamarta D, Aguas J, Ferrer E. The natural history of arachnoid cysts: endoscopic and cine-mode MRI evidence of a slit-valve mechanism. Minim Inv Neurosurg 1995;38(4):133−7.

[43] Schroeder HW, Gaab MR, Niendorf WR. Neuroendoscopic approach to arachnoid cysts. J Neurosurg 1996;85(2):293−8.

[44] Berle M, et al. Quantitative proteomics comparison of arachnoid cyst fluid and cerebrospinal fluid collected perioperatively from arachnoid cyst patients. Fluids Barriers CNS 2013;10(1):17.

[45] Berle M, et al. Arachnoid cysts do not contain cerebrospinal fluid: a comparative chemical analysis of arachnoid cyst fluid and cerebrospinal fluid in adults. Cerebrospinal Fluid Res 2010;7:8.

[46] Helland CA, et al. Increased NKCC1 expression in arachnoid cysts supports secretory basis for cyst formation. Exp Neurol 2010;224(2):424−8.

[47] Gelabert-Gonzalez M, et al. << De novo >> development of a suprasellar arachnoid cyst. Neurocirugia (Astur) 2015;26(2):100−4.

[48] Invergo D, Tomita T. De novo suprasellar arachnoid cyst: case report and review of the literature. Pediatr Neurosurg 2012;48(3):199−203.

[49] Kumagai M, et al. Postnatal development and enlargement of primary middle cranial fossa arachnoid cyst recognized on repeat CT scans. Childs Nerv Syst 1986;2(4): 211−15.

[50] Iglesias-Pais M, et al. De novo arachnoid cyst treated with a cystoperitoneal shunt. Rev Neurol 2003;36(12):1149−52.

[51] Struck AF, Murphy MJ, Iskandar BJ. Spontaneous development of a de novo suprasellar arachnoid cyst. Case report. J Neurosurg 2006;104(6 Suppl):426−8.

[52] Martinez-Lage JF, et al. Development of a middle fossa arachnoid cyst. A theory on its pathogenesis. Childs Nerv Syst 1999;15(2−3):94−7.

[53] Rao G, et al. Expansion of arachnoid cysts in children: report of two cases and review of the literature. J Neurosurg 2005;102(3 Suppl):314−17.

[54] Okumura Y, Sakaki T, Hirabayashi H. Middle cranial fossa arachnoid cyst developing in infancy. Case report. J Neurosurg 1995;82(6):1075−7.

[55] Mattei TA, et al. Benign extracerebral fluid collection in infancy as a risk factor for the development of de novo intracranial arachnoid cysts. J Neurosurg Pediatr 2013; 12(6):555−64.

[56] Lutcherath V, et al. Children with bilateral temporal arachnoid cysts may have glutaric aciduria type 1 (GAT1); operation without knowing that may be harmful. Acta Neurochir (Wien) 2000;142(9):1025−30.

[57] Alvarez LA, Maytal J, Shinnar S. Idiopathic external hydrocephalus-natural-history and relationship to benign familial macrocephaly. Pediatrics 1986;77(6):901−7.

[58] Laubscher B, et al. Primitive megalencephaly in children-natural-history, medium term prognosis with special reference to external hydrocephalus. Eur J Pediatr 1990;149(7):502−7.

[59] Muenchberger H, et al. Idiopathic macrocephaly in the infant: long-term neurological and neuropsychological outcome. Childs Nerv Syst 2006;22(10):1242−8.

[60] Prassopoulos P, et al. The size of the intraventricular and extraventricular cerebrospinal-fluid compartments in children with idiopathic benign widening of the frontal subarachnoid space. Neuroradiology 1995;37(5):418−21.

[61] Yew AY, et al. Long-term health status in benign external hydrocephalus. Pediatr Neurosurg 2011;47(1):1−6.

[62] Graillon T, et al. Adult symptomatic and growing arachnoid cyst successfully treated by ventriculocystostomy: a new insight on adult arachnoid cyst history. Neurochirurgie 2013;59(6):218−20.

[63] Halani SH, Safain MG, Heilman CB. Arachnoid cyst slit valves: the mechanism for arachnoid cyst enlargement. J Neurosurg Pediatr 2013;12(1):62−6.

[64] Kurabe S, et al. Growing posterior fossa arachnoid cyst causing tonsillar herniation and hydrocephalus. Arch Neurol 2011;68(12):1606−7.

[65] Wester K, Moen G. Documented growth of a temporal arachnoid cyst. J Neurol Neurosurg Psychiatry 2000;69(5):699−700.

[66] Al-Holou WN, et al. Prevalence and natural history of arachnoid cysts in adults. J Neurosurg 2013;118(2):222−31.

[67] Rabiei K, et al. Prevalence and symptoms of intracranial arachnoid cysts: a population-based study. J Neurol 2016;263(4):689−94.

[68] Vernooij MW, et al. Incidental findings on brain MRI in the general population. N Engl J Med 2007;357(18):1821−8.

[69] Weber F, Knopf H. Incidental findings in magnetic resonance imaging of the brains of healthy young men. J Neurol Sci 2006;240(1−2):81−4.

[70] Helland CA, Wester K. A population based study of intracranial arachnoid cysts: clinical and neuroimaging outcomes following surgical cyst decompression in adults. J Neurol Neurosurg Psychiatry 2007;78(10):1129−35.

[71] Helland CA, Wester K. Intracystic pressure in patients with temporal arachnoid cysts: a prospective study of preoperative complaints and postoperative outcome. J Neurol Neurosurg Psychiatry 2007;78(6):620−3.

[72] Morkve SH, et al. Surgical decompression of arachnoid cysts leads to improved quality of life: a prospective study. Neurosurgery 2016;78(5):613−25.

Arachnoid Cysts and Subdural and Intracystic Hematomas

Knut Wester[1,2]

[1]University of Bergen, Bergen, Norway
[2]Haukeland University Hospital, Bergen, Norway

OUTLINE

Arachnoid Cysts: Epidemiology, Biology, and Neuroimaging
DOI: http://dx.doi.org/10.1016/B978-0-12-809932-2.00012-0

ABBREVIATIONS

AC   arachnoid cyst
BEH   benign external hydrocephalus
BESS   benign enlargement of the subarachnoid spaces
CSDH   chronic subdural hematomas

INTRODUCTION

Patients harboring an arachnoid cyst (AC) are predisposed for chronic intracystic and subdural hematomas (CSDH); many of these patients appear to be in the younger half of the population, not infrequently also in children [1−4] (Fig. 12.1). To my knowledge, one of the first reports of an association between skull deformities as seen in children with AC and subdural hematomas was that of Bull in 1949 [5]. A decade earlier, Davidoff and Dyke had described a similar phenomenon, the "relapsing juvenile chronic subdural hematomas" [6], a terminology that no longer seems to be in use.

Chronic intracystic hematomas have also been reported in AC patients—together with CSDH [7] or as isolated intracystic hematomas [8] (Fig. 12.2). Almost an overwhelming number of reports on the association between AC and such chronic extracerebral hematomas have been published since the first reports (e.g., see [1−4,9−19]). Although both CSDH and AC are common in the general population, and simultaneity of the two conditions therefore might be incidental, this abundance of reports on the coexistence of AC and extracerebral hematomas indicate very strongly a causal relationship, most probably that an AC predisposes for such hematomas.

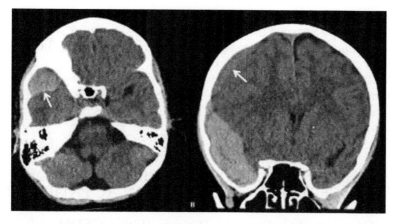

FIGURE 12.1 CT scan of an 8-year-old boy who sustained mild head trauma when playing soccer. He subsequently developed headaches. Left: axial scan; right: coronal scan, both showing hemorrhage into a relatively small right middle fossa AC (left—arrow) with extension into a right convexity subdural hematoma (right—arrow) with midline shift. *Printed with permission from Dr. J. Gordon McComb, see also Chapter 18, Pediatric Cranial Arachnoid Cysts, of Volume 2.*

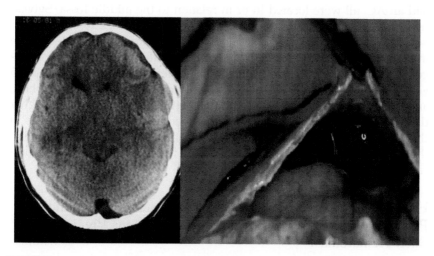

FIGURE 12.2 CT scan of an intracystic hematoma in a left middle fossa cyst without CSDH. Left: axial scan. Please note isodensity of the hematoma-filled cyst. Right: intraoperative photo of the same cyst, dark because of the intracystic hematoma. Please note the lack of subdural hematoma over the cortex.

The following seven questions will be asked and attempted to be answered in the present chapter:

1. What is the frequency/prevalence of extracerebral hematomas in AC patients?

2. Who are at risk of getting such spontaneous hematomas?
3. What are the possible mechanisms behind the bleeding?
4. How dangerous are spontaneous extracerebral hematomas in AC patients and what are the symptoms?
5. Which surgical procedures have been used?
6. Intracranial aneurysms and AC—is there an association?
7. Can extracerebral hematomas in AC patients be misinterpreted as having been caused by physical child abuse?

WHAT IS THE FREQUENCY/PREVALENCE OF EXTRACEREBRAL HEMATOMAS IN AC PATIENTS?

How Often are ACs Found in Patients With a CSDH and Where Are These Cyst Located?

Three reports have investigated the reverse association: how often an AC can be found in patients with a CSDH. In 658 patients between 5 and 80 years (mean 34 years) with CSDH, Parsch et al. found that 2.43% also had an AC, all were located in or in relation to the middle fossa/Sylvian fissure [3]. Mori et al. found a similar frequency: 12 (2.2%) of a total of 541 CSDH patients had an associated AC, two-thirds were located in the middle fossa [16]. Zheng et al. [19] investigated this association in a younger cohort of CSDH patients, a total of 45 patients in the age range 10–45 years. There was a marked male preponderance (93.3%) in this cohort, and the proportion that was associated with an AC was much higher than what was reported in the two other studies (11.1%). The five ACs in this study were all located in the middle fossa. Although investigating the reverse relationship, the three studies referred to above strongly indicate an association between AC and CSDH.

How Often Are Chronic Extracerebral Hematomas Found in Patients With an AC and Which Cyst Locations Predispose for Such Hematomas?

To my knowledge, only three reports have studied the frequency of extracerebral hematomas in patients harboring an AC. Galassi et al. [20] reported a total of 7 patients (9.1%) harboring a subdural or intracystic hematoma in a cohort of 77 patients harboring a middle fossa cyst.

Cress et al. found a hematoma frequency of 6.0% in 232 untreated AC patients [21]. The last study reporting on hematoma frequency was population based and included all consecutive AC patients that were referred to our department for a symptomatic AC [4]. The total number of patients was 241; 193 (80.1%) adults and 48 (19.9%) children. The majority of the patients (168) had a temporal cyst. For all the patients, neuroimaging had verified an AC, with or without a chronic hematoma. Most of the patients were operated, including all the patients with a hematoma. Thus, the presence of a hematoma in this study was verified both by neuroimaging and the subsequent operation. A total of 11 patients (4.6%; eight males and three females) were admitted because of a chronic hematoma (10 patients), or had been operated for a hematoma in another department prior to hospitalization in our department (one patient). None of the patients had a history of recurrent hematomas. The preoperative symptoms were combinations of headache, nausea, vertigo, fatigue, or cognitive impairment in eight patients. The remaining three patients also had impaired contralateral sensorimotor function. In seven patients, the hematoma was preceded by a distinct head trauma; the remaining four patients did not have any previous head trauma. Five patients had only a CSDH; the other six had both a CSDH and a chronic intracystic hematoma. The age of the hematoma patients varied between 2 years 5 months and 61 years (mean 28 years, median 23.5 years). Two of the patients were children; nine were adults. The age and gender did not differ from the other cyst patients. In this study, there was no difference in the hematoma frequency between small, middle sized, or large temporal cysts.

The CSDH and intracystic hematomas were found only in patients with temporal fossa cysts. As mentioned above: the frequency of hematomas for all cyst locations was 4.6%. However, as hematomas only occurred in patients with temporal fossa cysts, it may be more appropriate to look at the frequency for temporal cysts isolated: 6.5%. A literature survey that was performed for the same study [4] also revealed a disproportionately higher occurrence of hematomas for temporal fossa cysts than for cysts in any other location. Approximately two-thirds of ACs are located in the temporal fossa [22], but in this survey as many as 94 hematoma-associated cysts (90.4%) were located there; only 10 cysts (9.6%) were found in other locations. The impression that temporal cysts are disproportionately more prone to elicit chronic hematomas is further supported by a recent updated review of published cases; 37 of a total of 41 AC patients with hematomas had middle fossa cysts [14].

We have also learned from the first three studies referred to in this section that temporal fossa cysts appear more frequently in CSDH patients than cysts in other locations do. It therefore seems important to know the prevalence of hematomas for the middle fossa location. Galassi et al. studied temporal cysts only and found a hematoma frequency of 9.1%, not too different from the frequency we found for temporal cysts: 6.5%.

Should We Then Operate Arachnoid Cysts to Prevent the Development of Future Hematomas?

The studies referred in this chapter show that AC patients harbor a lifelong risk of incurring CSDH or intracystic hematomas as a complication to their cysts. It seems reasonable to view this risk as an indication for decompressive surgery in order to prevent future hematomas. However, the risk for suffering a spontaneous hematoma appears to be in the same order of magnitude as the risk of getting a subdural hematoma as a postoperative complication to cyst surgery [23,24]. Consequently, there seems to be little reason to operate a cyst with the sole purpose of preventing future hematomas.

WHO ARE AT RISK OF GETTING SPONTANEOUS HEMATOMAS ASSOCIATED WITH AN AC?

Age Doesn't Seem to Matter

As mentioned above, AC patients have a lifelong risk of sustaining CSDH or intracystic hematomas as a complication to their cysts. One might get the impression from the literature that children are more susceptible to such hematomas than adults; this impression is however most likely caused by a selection bias due to case studies or reviews on pure pediatric populations [14]. In our population-based study, we found CSDH and/or intracystic hematomas in 11 AC patients, with an age distribution that seemed to reflect that of the general population: two patients in each decade up to 50, and one above 60 [4]. Four other studies, reporting the experience from the authors' own departments, show a similar normal age distribution [2,3,10,16], and one review article also contained a substantial portion of adults [1].

In conclusion, chronic extracerebral hematomas associated with an AC appear not to be confined to any particular age group.

Does Gender Matter?

In all published reports on the topic, there is a male preponderance; this however seems to be of the same magnitude as the male prevalence for the most common location—the middle fossa. Thus, gender does not seem to be a parameter of importance for the risk of developing a CSDH or an intracystic hematoma.

Cyst Location—Middle Fossa Cysts Are Overrepresented in Patients With Extracerebral Hematomas

This factor is partly dealt with in the discussion above. It seems quite obvious from the data presented there that patients with a middle fossa AC are more prone to acquire a chronic extracerebral hematoma than patients with cysts anywhere else [1−4,14].

Does Cyst Size Matter?

Available data are rather scarce on this topic; to my knowledge, only three reports have looked at the importance of cyst size. In our study referred to above, there was no correlation between cyst size and hematoma frequency [4]. However, in the other patient-based study [21], with a similar patient cohort (232 vs 241), Cress et al. found that when dichotomized into larger and smaller cysts (with an arbitrarily set cut-off: maximal cyst diameter above or below 5 cm), the hematoma prevalence was significantly higher (9/13) in the larger cysts, than in the smaller ones (5/29).

Using a model of normal male adult head/brain, Lee et al. [25] calculated that the shearing forces for middle fossa cyst walls increased with increasing cyst size, thus giving some support to the findings reported by Cress et al. See also the following section.

Prior Head Injury

A head injury is quite often reported to have preceded the symptom debut by weeks or even months in a little more than a half of the patients. As most of these events were described as "mild" and as mild head injuries are not infrequent in the population, especially among children and young adults, it is difficult to take this as evidence for a causal relationship. What we do learn from the literature, however, is that a CSDH and/or an intracystic hematoma can occur without any preceding head trauma and that head traumas does not seem to cause acute and dramatic symptoms. See also Chapter 20 in Volume 2 on sport activities.

WHAT ARE THE POSSIBLE MECHANISMS BEHIND THE BLEEDING?

Normally, CSDH is almost exclusively found in elderly patients. When such hematomas occur in young adults and even in children with an AC, it is reasonable to assume a causal relationship between the two conditions.

So, what could be the underlying pathophysiological mechanisms? The loose attachment between the arachnoid and dura may be a part of the answer; in fact, the arachnoid apparently tears easily away from the dura when subjected to weak mechanical forces, e.g., when merely opening the dura during a surgical procedure.

The subdural compartment is probably regarded by most clinicians, neurosurgeons included [26], as a potential space between the inner layer of the dura mater and the outer layers of the arachnoid, much in the same way as the space formed by the two layers of the pleura. Anatomically, however, this is not the case [27–30]. On the contrary, there is a cellular continuity between the inner cell layer of the dura and the outer, barrier cell layer of the arachnoid. The so-called "subdural space" is thus not a normal anatomical cleavage, but a result of tissue damage—a dehiscence of the dural border cells.

We have during our operations for AC regularly observed how easily the parietal AC membrane, i.e., the cyst wall that lines the dural surface in the middle fossa, is detached from the dura. Just lowering the intracystic pressure by opening the cyst is often sufficient to cause the membrane to detach from the dura. When this occurs, multiple small vascular openings in the unveiled dura often begin to ooze blood. The loosely attached parietal cyst membrane thus seems to serve as an extra wall or support for these dural vascular structures. It is conceivable that the mechanical forces during a moderate head trauma can cause the cyst membrane to be detached from dura, thus initiating a bleeding episode. This mechanism may also explain why chronic hematomas also can be found in association with spinal ACs, reflecting the rather pronounced mechanical forces exerted during movements of the spine [31–35].

The second intraoperative observation of ours is along the same line. The parietal cyst membrane also covers the area where the bridging Sylvian veins, or the veins that traverse the cyst membrane unsupported by brain tissue, enter into the dural venous sinuses behind the sphenoid ridge. As long as the membrane is in normal contact with dura, these veins are supported by the arachnoid. If the parietal membrane is detached from the dura, which inevitably will happen during cyst decompression, the veins are no longer covered and supported by the arachnoid. This lack of support can induce leakage of blood into the subdural compartment from the entry point of these veins, as suggested by Page et al. [17]. It is also our experience that membranes of cysts in other locations—mostly frontal cysts on the convexity—do not cover dural vascular structures to the same extent. This may be a possible explanation for the disproportionately more frequent occurrence of hematomas associated with cysts in the temporal fossa, compared with cysts in other locations.

In this context, the report of Lee et al. is interesting. In their model study they showed increased shearing forces on the outer cyst wall compared with the normal brain when subjected to simulated "traumas" [25]. This observation may be relevant for both explanations of a subdural bleeding that are launched above—the oozing from the unveiled dural surface and from the bridging veins' entry into the dural sinuses. Shearing forces affecting the outside of the cyst wall may result in detachment of the arachnoid together with the innermost cell layer of dura.

HOW DANGEROUS ARE SPONTANEOUS EXTRACEREBRAL HEMATOMAS IN AC PATIENTS?

Spontaneous CSDH and chronic intracystic hematomas in AC patients usually have a gradual and slow symptom onset that rarely necessitates urgent surgery. In most high-income countries, where neurosurgical service is easily available, such hematomas can therefore be regarded as relatively low-risk complications to an AC. However, they may represent more severe problems in countries with less developed or scarce neurosurgical facilities. As all reports on AC associated hematomas come from countries with reasonably well developed medical institutions, the available information on symptoms and severity comes from patients that have been adequately treated. That applies also to clinical outcome, which in general is reported as good.

In nine case series [1,3,4,10,14,16−19] that give detailed reports on symptoms and symptom severity in more than one patient, comprising a total of 68 patients, headache, nausea, and vomiting were the most common symptoms. In addition, hemisphere related symptoms, mostly mild hemipareses, were seen in 17 patients, three patients complained of disturbed vision, and two had seizures. Reduced consciousness was not described in these reports, but a few elderly suffered a mild confusion.

WHICH SURGICAL PROCEDURES HAVE BEEN USED?

For ACs associated with chronic extracerebral hematomas, two surgical options have been used: burr hole with evacuation/irrigation of the CSDH only; or craniotomy with evacuation of the CSDH and simultaneous extirpation/fenestration of the cyst. From the literature, it seems as if the choice of method is based solely on the beliefs and preference of the surgeon, not on evidence. In our series [4], we preferred the latter method and had good results, but good outcome was also reported for those that only evacuated the hematoma and left the cyst untouched [16,19] or for those that used both methods [36]. Thus, there is no clear-cut indication in the literature to what is the best method.

INTRACRANIAL ANEURYSMS AND AC - IS THERE AN ASSOCIATION?

There seems to be an association between intracranial aneurysms and AC. At least 16 publications were identified in a literature search ("arachnoid cyst* AND aneurysm") [9,37–51]. Both conditions have relatively high prevalence in the population, but the large number of reports on this unusual combination nevertheless indicates a nonincidental correlation. All ACs that have been described in association with aneurysms have been located in the middle fossa.

The onset is of course abrupt if the aneurysm ruptures, but if the bleeding is confined to the cyst cavity, the symptoms may not be as dramatic as in an ordinary subarachnoid hemorrhage (SAH), and the cerebrospinal fluid may even be clear [40,41,47,50]. On the other hand, the clinical picture may also be as dramatic as after an SAH, death may even occur [9].

Most cases have been diagnosed after rupture of an aneurysm dome that bulges into the cyst cavity; it is reasonable to assume that the dome ruptures more easily through a thin cyst wall than if it is supported by overlying, solid brain tissue. Maybe this is the explanation of the apparent correlation; both conditions are relatively common and when they by incidence coexist, the aneurysm bursts more easily because of the lack of support/resistance from its surroundings.

CAN EXTRACEREBRAL HEMATOMAS IN AC PATIENTS BE MISINTERPRETED AS HAVING BEEN CAUSED BY PHYSICAL CHILD ABUSE?

It is relatively well known that Benign External Hydrocephalus (BEH—also called BESS and other names) predisposes for both chronic and acute SDH, often of different ages. As the finding of SDH in a child almost automatically causes the involved health personnel to suspect physical child abuse ("shaken baby syndrome"), BEH may represent a dangerous pitfall in the subsequent work-up of the child [52].

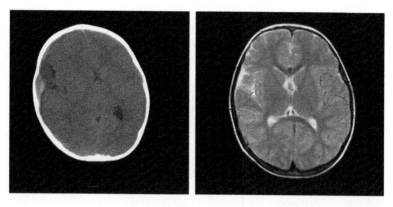

FIGURE 12.3 Left: preoperative axial CT scan showing a peripheral CSDH and an intracystic hematoma. Right: MRI 3 months after evacuation of the hematomas and fenestration of the cyst. *Reproduced from Wester K, Helland CA. How often do chronic extra-cerebral haematomas occur in patients with intracranial arachnoid cysts? JNNP 2008;79:72–75 [4]. With permission from BMJ Publishing Group Ltd.*

It is not so well known that an AC-induced CSDH can be misinterpreted in the same way. Such cases have not been reported in the literature, but I have personally witnessed health personnel that were convinced of child abuse in a 2.4-year-old girl with a temporal fossa AC and CSDHs of different ages, see Fig. 12.3.

Thus, in order to avoid such mistakes that may be devastating to the family, it is important to be aware of the possibility that the child may have an AC as the underlying cause of the hematomas.

References

[1] Bilginer B, et al. Arachnoid cyst associated with subdural hematoma: report of three cases and review of the literature. Childs Nerv Syst 2009;25(1):119–24.
[2] Iaconetta G, et al. Arachnoid cyst with intracystic haemorrhage and subdural haematoma: case report and literature review. Neurol Sci 2006;26(6):451–5.
[3] Parsch CS, et al. Arachnoid cysts associated with subdural hematomas and hygromas: analysis of 16 cases, long-term follow-up, and review of the literature. Neurosurgery 1997;40(3):483–90.
[4] Wester K, Helland CA. How often do chronic extra-cerebral haematomas occur in patients with intracranial arachnoid cysts? J Neurol Neurosurg Psychiatry 2008;79(1): 72–5.
[5] Bull JW. The diagnosis of chronic subdural haematoma in children and adolescents. Br J Radiol 1949;22(254):68–80.
[6] Davidoff LM, Dyke CG. Relapsing juvenile chronic subdural haematomas. Bull Neurol Instit 1938;7:95–111.
[7] Romero FJ, et al. Arachnoid cysts with intracystic and subdural-hematoma. Eur J Radiol 1989;9(2):119–20.
[8] Ildan F, et al. Arachnoid cyst with traumatic intracystic hemorrhage unassociated with subdural-hematoma. Neurosurg Rev 1994;17(3):229–32.

[9] Burke MP, O'Donnell C, Opeskin K. Spontaneous acute subdural hematoma complicating arachnoid cyst. Am J Forensic Med Pathol 2010;31(4):382–4.

[10] Domenicucci M, et al. Relationship between supratentorial arachnoid cyst and chronic subdural hematoma: neuroradiological evidence and surgical treatment. J Neurosurg 2009;110(6):1250–5.

[11] Henriques JG, et al. Spontaneous acute subdural hematoma contralateral to an arachnoid cyst. Arq Neuropsiquiatr 2007;65(4A):1034–6.

[12] Islamian AP, Polemikos M, Krauss JK. Chronic subdural haematoma secondary to headbanging. Lancet 2014;384(9937). p. 102.

[13] Kobayashi A, et al. A case of organized arachnoid cyst with repeated hemorrhage. Clin Case Rep 2016;4(3):250–4.

[14] Liu Z, et al. Arachnoid cysts with subdural hematoma or intracystic hemorrhage in children. Pediatr Emerg Care 2014;30(5):345–51.

[15] Maeda M, et al. Value of Mr-imaging in middle fossa arachnoid cyst with intracystic and subdural-hematoma. Eur J Radiol 1993;17(3):145–7.

[16] Mori K, et al. Arachnoid cyst is a risk factor for chronic subdural hematoma in juveniles: twelve cases of chronic subdural hematoma associated with arachnoid cyst. J Neurotr 2002;19(9):1017–27.

[17] Page A, Paxton RM, Mohan D. A reappraisal of the relationship between arachnoid cysts of the middle fossa and chronic subdural haematoma. J Neurol Neurosurg Psychiatry 1987;50(8):1001–7.

[18] Servadei F, et al. Arachnoid cyst of middle cranial fossa and ipsilateral subdural haematoma: diagnostic and therapeutic implications in three cases. Br J Neurosurg 1993;7(3):249–53.

[19] Zheng SP, Li GP, You C. Chronic subdural hematoma associated with arachnoid cysts in young people. Neurosurg Quart 2013;23(4):258–61.

[20] Galassi E, et al. Arachnoid cysts of the middle cranial fossa: experience with 77 cases treated surgically. Acta Neurochir Suppl (Wien) 1988;42:201–4.

[21] Cress M, et al. Risk factors for pediatric arachnoid cyst rupture/hemorrhage: a case-control study. Neurosurgery 2013;72(5):716–22 discussion 722.

[22] Helland CA, Lund-Johansen M, Wester K. Location, sidedness, and sex distribution of intracranial arachnoid cysts in a population-based sample. J Neurosurg 2010;113(5):934–9.

[23] Helland CA, Wester K. A population based study of intracranial arachnoid cysts: clinical and neuroimaging outcomes following surgical cyst decompression in adults. J Neurol Neurosurg Psychiatry 2007;78(10):1129–35.

[24] Morkve SH, et al. Surgical decompression of arachnoid cysts leads to improved quality of life: a prospective study. Neurosurgery 2016;78(5):613–25.

[25] Lee CH, et al. Analysis of a bleeding mechanism in patients with the sylvian arachnoid cyst using a finite element model. Childs Nerv Syst 2014;30(6):1029–36.

[26] Penfield WG. The cranial subdural space: a method of study. Anatom Rec 1924;28:173–5.

[27] Haines DE. On the question of a subdural space. Anatom Rec 1991;230(1):3–21.

[28] Haines DE, Harkey HL, al-Mefty O. The "subdural" space: a new look at an outdated concept. Neurosurgery 1993;32(1):111–20.

[29] Orlin JR, Osen KK, Hovig T. Subdural compartment in pig-a morphological-study with blood and horseradish-peroxidase infused subdurally. Anatom Rec 1991;230(1):22–37.

[30] Schachenmayr W, Friede RL. The origin of subdural neomembranes. I. Fine structure of the dura-arachnoid interface in man. Am J Pathol 1978;92(1):53–68.

[31] Fobe JL, Nishikuni K, Gianni MA. Evolving magnetic resonance spinal cord trauma in child: from hemorrhage to intradural arachnoid cyst. Spinal Cord 1998;36(12):864–6.

[32] Kang HS, Chung CK, Kim HJ. Spontaneous spinal subdural hematoma with spontaneous resolution. Spinal Cord 2000;38(3):192–6.

[33] Muthukumar N. Anterior cervical arachnoid cyst presenting with traumatic quadriplegia. Childs Nerv Syst 2004;20(10):757–60.

[34] Spiegelmann R, Rappaport ZH, Sahar A. Spinal arachnoid cyst with unusual presentation. Case report. J Neurosurg 1984;60(3):613–16.

[35] Teruel Agustin JJ, et al. Computed tomography of a post traumatic spinal arachnoid cyst. Neuroradiology 1989;31(4):354–5.

[36] Sprung C, et al. Arachnoid cysts of the middle cranial fossa accompanied by subdural effusions–experience with 60 consecutive cases. Acta Neurochir (Wien) 2011;153(1):75–84 discussion 84.

[37] Barker RA, et al. Posterior communicating artery aneurysm presenting with haemorrhage into an arachnoid cyst. J Neurol Neurosurg Psychiatry 1998;64(4):558–60.

[38] Baykal S, et al. Aneurysm of an azygos anterior cerebral artery: report of two cases and review of the literature. Neurosurg Rev 1996;19(1):57–9.

[39] de Oliveira JG, et al. Intracranial aneurysm and arachnoid cyst: a rare association between two cerebral malformations. Br J Neurosurg 2007;21(4):406–10.

[40] Hirose S, et al. Ruptured aneurysm associated with arachnoid cyst: intracystic hematoma without subarachnoid hemorrhage. Surg Neurol 1995;43(4):353–6.

[41] Huang D, et al. Intracystic hemorrhage of the middle fossa arachnoid cyst and subdural hematoma caused by ruptured middle cerebral artery aneurysm. AJNR Am J Neuroradiol 1999;20(7):1284–6.

[42] Jinkins JR, Siqueira EB, Holoubi A. Ruptured middle cerebral aneurysm with accumulation of subarachnoid blood within convexity arachnoid cyst. Comput Radiol 1987;11(4):185–7.

[43] Kajiwara I, et al. Intracystic hematoma of middle fossa arachnoid cyst caused by rupture of internal carotid-posterior communicating artery aneurysm. Neurol Med Chir (Tokyo) 2008;48(5):220–2.

[44] Kocaeli H, Korfali E. Rupture of a small middle cerebral artery aneurysm into middle fossa arachnoid cyst presenting as a chronic subdural haematoma. Acta Neurochir (Wien) 2008;150(4):407–8.

[45] Leo JS, et al. Computed tomography of arachnoid cysts. Radiology 1979;130(3):675–80.

[46] Secer HI, et al. Endoscopic clipping of a middle cerebral artery aneurysm in a middle fossa arachnoid cyst and review of the literature. Minim Inv Neurosurg 2010;53(3):132–7.

[47] Shimizu J, et al. An aneurysm rupturing into a middle cranial fossa arachnoid cyst presenting as an intracystic hemorrhage. J Stroke Cerebrovasc Dis 2012;21(3):243–4.

[48] Sun T, Zhao J. Multiple saccular aneurysms of the extracranial and intracranial internal carotid artery associated with convexobasia and arachnoid cyst in a 6-year-old boy: a case report. Childs Nerv Syst 2010;26(1):113–16.

[49] Schumacher M, Baust W, Terwey B. Unusual combination of cerebral dysplasias - report of 2 cases. Neurochirurgia 1986;29(5):210–14.

[50] Trivelato FP, et al. Endovascular treatment of a traumatic carotid artery aneurysm after endoscopic arachnoid cyst fenestration. Childs Nerv Syst 2011;27(8):1329–32.

[51] Zanini MA, et al. A form of dysplasia or a fortuitous association? A cerebral aneurysm inside an arachnoid cyst: case report. Neurosurgery 2007;61(3):E654–5 discussion E655.

[52] Gabaeff SC. Exploring the controversy in child abuse pediatrics and false accusations of abuse. Legal Med 2016;18:90–7.

CHAPTER

13

Hydrocephalus Associated With Arachnoid Cysts

Juan F. Martínez-Lage[1,2], Claudio Piqueras[1,2] and María-José Almagro[1]

[1]Virgen de la Arrixaca University Hospital, Murcia, Spain
[2]University of Murcia Medical School, Murcia, Spain

OUTLINE

Arachnoid Cysts: Epidemiology, Biology, and Neuroimaging
DOI: http://dx.doi.org/10.1016/B978-0-12-809932-2.00013-2

139

ABBREVIATIONS

AC	arachnoid cyst
CSF	cerebrospinal fluid
CP	cystoperitoneal (shunt)
CT	computerized tomography
EEG	electroencephalography
ETV	endoscopic third ventriculostomy
ICP	intracranial pressure
MRI	magnetic resonance imaging
PET	positron emission tomography
SPECT	single-photon emission computed tomography
US	ultrasonography
VP	ventriculoperitoneal (shunt)

INTRODUCTION

Bright is credited for the first description of an arachnoid cyst (AC). He also suggested that these pouches were "serous cysts forming in connection with the arachnoid and apparently lying *between* its layers" (Bright, 1831, see Chapter 1, Arachnoid Cysts—Historical Perspectives and Controversial Aspects). Arachnoid pouches were initially described under the names of *meningitis serosa circumscripta, chronic arachnoiditis,* or *cerebral pseudotumor.* Due to the limited information that the initial diagnostic methods could supply, early reports of intracranial ACs almost always corresponded to highly symptomatic patients and to those evolving with hydrocephalus [1–3]. The advent of the current neuroimaging methods, such as computerized tomography (CT) and magnetic resonance imaging (MRI), contributed to a better understanding of the natural history of ACs.

An AC consists of a cavity filled with a fluid similar in composition to cerebrospinal fluid (CSF). The cyst's walls are lined by arachnoid cells and abundant veins. ACs are typically situated within the split arachnoid membrane, hence they are truly intraarachnoid. The theory of the temporal lobe agenesis for explaining the origin of ACs has practically been abandoned [1].

Most ACs are of *congenital* origin, although some of these pouches are considered to be *acquired*. In this case, there is a known antecedent of trauma, hemorrhage, inflammation, or tumor, and they may even be of iatrogenic origin [4–6]. Due to the widespread utilization of CT and MRI, many cysts are now detected during the diagnostic workup of unrelated conditions and are termed *incidental* ACs. The majority of incidentally discovered ACs produce no symptoms and require no surgical treatment [6,7].

In contrast, many patients with ACs are brought to consultation for clinical manifestations of raised intracranial pressure (ICP) or for symptoms related with the mass effect of the lesion. During the evaluation of symptomatic patients with ACs, the neuroimaging studies may show *ventriculomegaly* that apparently produce no brain damage. On the contrary, some individuals evolve with overt manifestations of *hydrocephalus*. Current studies have mainly documented the focal effects of ACs on the brain, but the consequences of AC-associated hydrocephalus seem to have received less attention. In this chapter, we will focus on the role of hydrocephalus in the context of ACs, discussing the origin and the diverse management options in the cases diagnosed with both conditions.

Reviewed articles possess a Level of Evidence IV or V.

MATERIAL AND METHODS

The content of the present chapter is based on a selection of key publications on ACs, and is mainly constituted by analysis of patients' series and some case-report papers. To address the goals of our chapter, we preferentially reviewed those publications dealing with the occurrence of hydrocephalus in patients with ACs. We also paid attention to those works that reported ACs-associated hydrocephalus in lesions situated in diverse locations, specially centering on the analysis of the various reported modalities of treatment. In certain cases we also included some data from our own experience that will not be discussed in detail in the present work.

EMBRYOPATHOGENESIS OF AC-RELATED HYDROCEPHALUS

An AC consists of an encapsulated pocket that contains a CSF-like fluid and whose walls are lined by arachnoid cells, veins, and collagen tissue. The name *arachnoid* derivates from the classic Greek word that means *spider* and refers to the web of fine threads constructed by a spider from fluid secreted by its spinnerets used to catch its prey. Since the initial description of Bright in 1831, ACs have been recognized as being truly intraarachnoid in location and thought to arise from a duplication of the arachnoid. The intraarachnoid nature of the ACs was later confirmed by microscopic and ultramicroscopic studies and by postmortem examinations.

During the early embryonic period, a loose layer of primitive mesenchyme, known as primitive meninx or endomeninx, wraps the neural tube. The endomeninx is believed to be the precursor of the pia- and arachnoid-matter. ACs develop about week 15 of gestation, when the subarachnoid layer is first identified. Following rhombic roof rupture, the CSF starts to circulate within this primitive subarachnoid space. Thus, the CSF dissects the arachnoid space and contributes to the development of the arachnoid, giving it a "web" disposition of delicate trabeculae.

Once the AC is formed, it can enlarge, decrease, or remain unchanged in size. The ACs can also arise "de novo" or they may even disappear either spontaneously or after trauma [8,9], see Chapter 11, Growth and Disappearance of Arachnoid Cysts. The expansion of an AC has been attributed to one of the following mechanisms: (1) the production of fluid by secretory cells that line the inner cyst walls; (2) the existence of an osmotic gradient between the cyst contents and the extracystic fluid; or (3) a ball-valve mechanism that allows the entry of CSF fluid within the cyst but that prevents its escape [6,10], see also Chapter 8, The "Valve Mechanism".

ACs and the Subarachnoid Spaces

The communication of ACs with the arachnoid space and basal cisterns has been documented by CT metrizamide-cisternography or by isotopic studies [11]. The ball-valve hypothesis has been verified in-vivo by cine mode-MRI and by direct observation during neuroendoscopy [10]. Even so, there also exists the possibility of the combined action of two or more of the abovementioned mechanisms in AC development.

Classically, ACs are classified into *communicating* and *noncommunicating*, referring to the relationship between the cyst's contents and the subarachnoid space. Galassi et al. [43] on reporting 31 cases of middle fossa ACs, described the findings of seven patients who were investigated by metrizamide CT cisternography and proposed a classification into three types (see also Chapter 10, Classification and Location of Arachnoid Cysts):

1. Type I refers to small, spindle-shaped lesions limited to the anterior aspect of the temporal fossa that usually do not produce a significant mass effect. In Type I middle fossa ACs, the lesions filled rapid and

massively with metrizamide indicating a free communication between the cyst and the subarachnoid spaces.

2. Galassi type II cysts are somewhat larger than Type I lesions. They have a triangular or quadrangular shape and produce some mass effect. They fill and drain in a delayed way compared to Type I cysts. A striking feature of Type II cysts is a metrizamide staining of some cortical subarachnoid spaces that surround the AC.

3. Type III ACs are the largest ones, oval or round in shape, that split the sylvian fissure. They produce a considerable mass effect and displace the ventricles and midline structures contralaterally. The fontal and parietal lobes appear severely compressed and there may be temporal lobe atrophy. They show no clear filling during metrizamide-cisternography indicating that these cysts have no communication with the subarachnoid space. However, there is some early and late metrizamide staining in the arachnoid spaces that surround the cyst. This feature seems to indicate that there exists a separation between the cyst and the underlying subarachnoid space and some CSF stasis in these spaces [43].

Unfortunately, these observations on the communication of sylvian ACs have not been investigated for ACs in other locations. However, one may hypothesize that other ACs must follow a similar pattern in regard to cyst–subarachnoid space connections.

Pathogenesis of AC-Associated Hydrocephalus

Several theories have been put forward to explain the occurrence of hydrocephalus in connection with ACs (Table 13.1):

1. *Compression and/or distortion of critical zones of the CSF pathways.* It is obvious that hydrocephalus can be produced by displacement/ compression of CSF pathways. This is especially true for ACs

TABLE 13.1 Theories on the Development of Hydrocephalus Associated With ACs

Theory
Compression of CSF pathways
Obstruction to CSF flow
Primary abnormality of CSF dynamics
Common origin for hydrocephalus and arachnoid cyst development
Diffuse secondary faulty development of the subarachnoid space and cerebral cisterns
Arachnoid cyst pressure on the cerebellar tonsils causing tonsillar descent/ hydrocephalus/ syringomyelia

occurring at critical sites. Hydrocephalus is more often found in instances of midline and posterior fossa ACs due to their proximity with the narrowest parts of the ventricular system. Suprasellar ACs may obstruct one or both foramina of Monro or compress the anterior third ventricle [6,12]. Cysts in or by the third ventricle, quadrigeminal region, or posterior fossa may distort or compress the CSF flow through the aqueduct of Sylvius [6,14]. ACs located at the posterior cranial fossa may directly compress the fourth ventricle foramina or may trap these orifices at the foramen magnum [13,14]. Hydrocephalus in intraventricular ACs is probably due to an obstruction in the lateral ventricle together with the intracystic accumulation of CSF that merges around the choroid plexus vessels [18].

2. *Primary abnormality of CSF dynamics.* Some authors suggest that the development of intracranial ACs and that of the associated hydrocephalus are intimately related and that it is due to impairment in CSF circulation or absorption [15,16]. An interesting hypothesis put forward the existence of preexisting hydrocephalus in the development of ACs. Patients initially diagnosed with arrested hydrocephalus later developed a middle fossa AC while the previously enlarged ventricles decreased in size in a similar way to that of communicating vessels [9].

A mechanism resembling external hydrocephalus (or benign pericerebral fluid collections) might also account for the formation of an AC as a compartmentalized form of hydrocephalus [17–19]. The entry of CSF would cause a dissection of the subarachnoid space forming a pouch that subsequently would become partially entrapped by a yet undefined mechanism (Figs. 13.1A–13.4A,B).

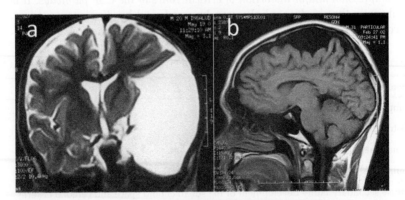

FIGURE 13.1 (A) Huge frontotemporal arachnoid cyst that displaces midline structures. Note enlarged pericerebral collections and skull asymmetry with bulging of the left hemicranium (reprinted with permission from Springer-Verlag). (B) Parietal convexity AC, note focal skull thinning and enlarged paranasal sinuses.

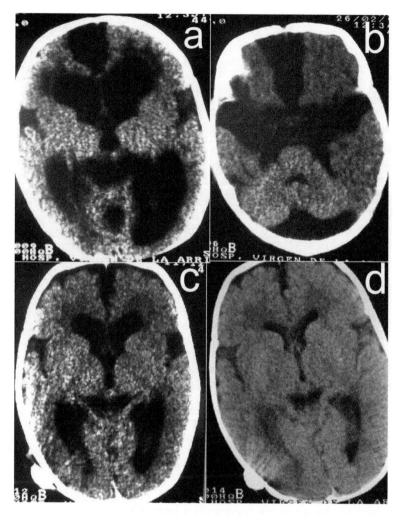

FIGURE 13.2   (A, B) CT images of an infant initially given a VP shunt showing multiple ACs and hydrocephalus; (C) decrease in size of the ventricles and cysts 6-months after VP shunting; (D) CT scan at age 3-year showing complete resolution of the hydrocephalus and cysts after VP shunting alone.

This theory would be sustained by the fact of an existing ample communication between the cysts and the subarachnoid space. In the same way, some of these cysts may completely disappear after ventriculoperitoneal (VP) shunting alone, which directly drains the cysts (Fig. 13.2). Consequently, ACs would represent *focal non-reabsorbtive hydrocephalus* (Fig. 13.1B) [17,18]. In a series of 40 patients with middle fossa ACs, there were six instances with hydrocephalus and nine with macrocephaly, suggesting that macrocephaly without

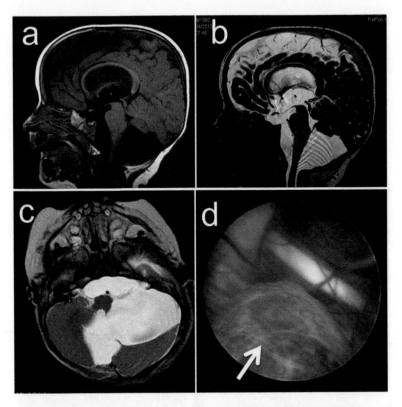

FIGURE 13.3   Posterior fossa and prepontine AC in an 5-month-old girl: (A) sagittal MRI showing a huge posterior fossa cyst and pericerebral fluid collections; (B) FIESTA sequences showing the retrocerebellar and prepontine cyst; (C) axial cut of MRI showing the extension of the AC; (D) endoscopic view of the cyst after puncture. The cyst was treated through a posterior fossa burr-hole combined with an endoscopic third ventriculostomy.

hydrocephalus probably represents a latent CSF circulation abnormality [20].

The appealing hypothesis of Mattei et al. [19] relates AC formation to preexisting benign extracerebral collections of fluid (Figs. 13.1A, 13.3A,B,C, and 13.4A,B). In a series of 44 children with benign extracerebral collections of infancy, 18 children (40.9%) developed de novo intracranial ACs, which were bilateral in 27.8% [19]. This theory, named as *the 2-hit hypothesis*, proposes the existence of a congenital defect in the embryological development of the arachnoid and a secondary event leading to impairment of intracranial CSF dynamics. These authors reported the presence of plagiocephaly and of bilateral frontal collections as risk factors for the formation of ACs [19], see also Chapter 11, Growth and Disappearance of Arachnoid

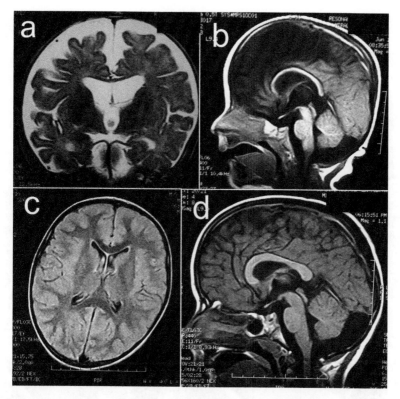

FIGURE 13.4   MRI of a 18-month-old-boy with a retrocerebellar cyst: (A) coronal view showing external hydrocephalus and ventricular enlargement; (B) sagittal view; (C) resolution of the pericerebral collections at age 3 years; (D) with unchanged posterior fossa cyst.

Cysts. In summary, the primary event would consist of a delay in the absorption of CSF that would increase the volume of pericerebral fluid that would, in turn, dissect a cavity within the arachnoid leading to the development of an AC. These events would be favored by the normal pulsating movements of the CSF and by the plasticity of the growing children' skull.

3. *Common pathogenesis of hydrocephalus and ACs.* Cysts arising in the interhemispheric fissure are often associated with hydrocephalus (Fig. 13.5). These cysts may or may not communicate with the ventricles, especially when they present with callosal dysgenesis (Fig. 13.6A,B). In one of our cases an intraventricular cyst became evident at the time of intracystic bleeding that occurred years after initial VP shunting (Fig. 13.6C).

4. *Secondary diffuse faulty development of the subarachnoid space.* In rare occasions hydrocephalus may coexist with bilateral (or multiple) cysts and their origin may be traced to a diffuse faulty development

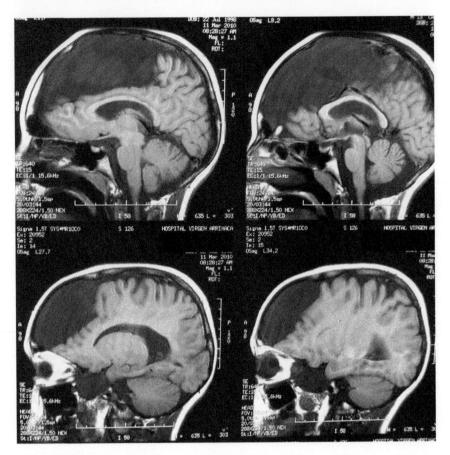

FIGURE 13.5   MRI performed to a 10-year-old boy with occasional headaches showing a frontoparietal interhemispheric AC. Note the integrity of the corpus callosum.

of the subarachnoid space as occurs in certain inherited disorders, such as neurofibromatosis or achondroplasia, and other conditions that evolve with cyst formation or with abnormal deposits in the subarachnoid space or in the cerebral convexities as occurs in glutaric aciduria type I [21–24], see also Chapter 4, Arachnoid Cysts in Glutaric Acidura Type I (GA-I).

5. *Cerebellar tonsils herniation and syringomyelia.* ACs in diverse locations of the posterior fossa may produce hydrocephalus, tonsillar descent (the so-called acquired Chiari anomaly) and syringomyelia [23,25]. Although its occurrence in ACs is very rare, tonsillar descent and associated syrinx constitute a main indication for surgery. There are two main mechanisms for explaining this event. In the first one, the cyst itself obstructs the foramen magnum and leads to the formation of a syrinx [26]. In the second one, the posterior fossa AC pushes the

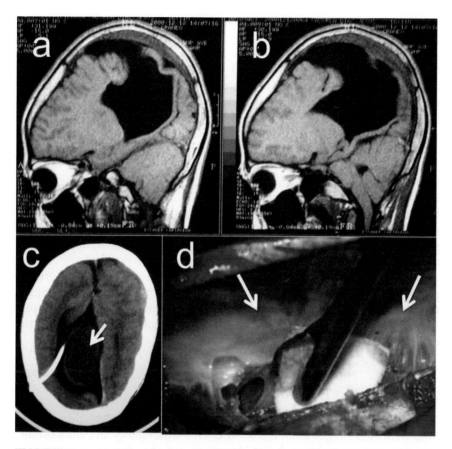

FIGURE 13.6   (A, B) Sagittal views of MRI showing an interhemispheric arachnoid cyst with corpus callosum dysgenesis and anomalous gyri in a child initially operated with a VP in the neonatal period; (C) intracystic hemorrhage at age 16 years; (D) photograph of the thick cyst membranes during craniotomy.

cerebellum within the foramen magnum and, by obstructing the up-and-down CSF movements at the craniovertebral junction, contributes to the development of hydrocephalus and syringomyelia [13,27].

EPIDEMIOLOGICAL DATA OF ACs WITH HYDROCEPHALUS

Arachnoid Cyst Overview

In the European Cooperative Study of ACs in children, ACs accounted for 1% of all intracranial space occupying lesions [50]. In a series of systematic necropsy examinations, the incidence was 5 per 5000 [50].

However, these figures must represent an underestimate as the Swedish population-based study gave a prevalence rate of ACs of 2.3% [28]. In a study of 209 symptomatic patients with ACs, 170 (81.3%) corresponded to patients in pediatric age and the remaining 39 were adults [29].

In addition, the advent of CT and MRI lead to the discovery of *incidental ACs* whose prevalence is presently unknown. In several series, ACs are more prevalent among males, exceeding females by a ratio of nearly 2:1 especially in middle fossa ACs [6,20,25,30]. Although ACs may present in all ages, most instances of AC manifest clinically during the first two decades of life with a mean age of 3.6 years in children and of 6 years in the European Cooperative Study [6,50]. Larger ACs that produce mass effect and those causing macrocephaly or hydrocephalus are more prevalent in younger ages.

Incidental ACs may also be discovered in any age. In a German population-based survey with emphasis on asymptomatic pathologies (incidental), ACs accounted for 7 of 3000 studies representing 2.3 per 1000 [31]. In another survey of 11,738 patients undergoing MRI, the rate of incidental ACs was of 309 (2.6%) [25].

Arachnoid Cyst-Related Hydrocephalus

According to diverse studies the incidence of hydrocephalus associated with ACs ranges from 2% to 80%. This discrepancy depends on the variable rate of hydrocephalus described for the diverse locations of ACs. In addition, initial publications refer to a higher rate of hydrocephalus in the context of intracranial ACs, probably due to the lesser resolution of available diagnostic methods of the epoch. Harrison reported hydrocephalus in 14 patients (100%) with ACs [3]. Marinov et al. [32] reported hydrocephalus in 2/3 of 58 children with ACs, all of them at the midline or the posterior fossa. Sommer and Smit [33] also documented hydrocephalus in 6 of 19 giant supratentorial ACs. Hydrocephalus was also present in 5 of 27 ACs reported by Rabiei et al. [28].

In a series of 309 ACs, hydrocephalus represented only 2.2% of the cases [25]. Galarza et al. [34] documented hydrocephalus in 7 of 33 children with ACs that corresponded to midline and to Galassi type III cysts. In the series of Fewell et al. [35] of 95 children with ACs, the rate of hydrocephalus was of 40%. A higher proportion of hydrocephalus was found in infratentorial ACs, 7 of 10 patients [36]. In a report comprising 170 children with ACs, all suprasellar ($n = 34$) and all ($n = 11$)

quadrigeminal cysts produced hydrocephalus [29]. The rate of hydro-cephalus is also very high in suprasellar ACs, reaching in diverse publi-cations the number of 100% (5 of 5) [37], 80% (16 of 20) [38], and 71% (5 of 7) [12], respectively. In a survey of quadrigeminal ACs, 14 of 14 (100%) cases evolved with obstructive hydrocephalus [39]. In purely intraparenchymal ACs, the hydrocephalus rate was 3 of 12 (25%) [40].

Regarding *prenatal* behavior of ACs, 54 fetuses were diagnosed prena-tally with intracranial cystic lesions, but only nine (16.6%) had ventriculo-megaly and only one (1.8%) developed progressive hydrocephalus [41].

Significance of Macrocephaly in ACs

Macrocephaly defines a larger than normal growth of the head with-out specifying a determined cause. Macrocephaly without hydrocepha-lus appears in many publications on ACs. For example, a recent work documented macrocephaly in a series of 27 ACs [28]. This association deserves some explanation.

In the study of Pascual-Castroviejo et al. [23] macrocephaly was the earliest and commonest mode of presentation of primary intracranial ACs, which occurred in 48 (71.5%) patients. Levy et al. [20] reported 40 children with middle fossa ACs and included six with hydrocephalus and nine with *nonspecific macrocephaly* (without ventriculomegaly). In their experience, all individuals presenting with hydrocephalus required a VP shunt in addition to open surgical fenestration of the cysts, regardless of which procedure had been performed first [20]. In addition, five patients with macrocephaly initially submitted to cyst fen-estration later required shunt placement, in contrast with the fact of that among 25 normocephalic children submitted to cyst fenestration only one required a CSF shunt [20].

In a survey of 111 ACs in all localizations, hydrocephalus was present in seven (2.2%) instances, eight patients developed progressive macroce-phaly, one developed increasing tonsillar descent with a cervical syrinx, and four exhibited symptoms and signs of increased ICP [25].

These publications suggest that macrocephaly in these patients repre-sent a *latent abnormality in CSF dynamics* similar to the mechanisms held responsible for the production of pseudotumor cerebri or of benign familial macrocephaly. Both extra-axial collections of infancy and pseu-dotumor cerebri might represent two different manifestations of the same process involving venous obstruction with decreased CSF absorp-tion and that they would manifest differently in children and adults [42]. Recent theories on the evolution of CSF dynamics have empha-sized the relevance of the so-called "minor pathways" (such as the dural plexus, subependymal venous pathways, the leptomeningeal to cortical veins and the pia-arachnoid-capillary routes, the choroid plexus capillary, and the perineural spaces pathways) for CSF drainage, especially in the first two years of life, when the arachnoid granulations have not yet fully developed [42]. Damage of these alternative pathways due to inflammation, trauma, or bleeding may lead to the accumulation of fluid in the subarachnoid spaces [42]. Accordingly, the initial event for AC development would consist of an non-reabsorbtive form of hydrocephalus (external hydrocephalus).

This attractive theory on macrocephaly with benign pericerebral collections for explaining the origin of ACs was put forward after a survey of pediatric patients evaluated by CT [19]. Interestingly, 18 of 44 (40.9%) children developed "de novo" ACs, some of them were multiple or bilateral. The authors propose that these extracerebral collections might play an important role in the formation of some ACs (Figs. 13.1A, 13.3A–C, and 13.4A,B), an opinion that we also advanced in a previous publication [18,19].

Hydrocephalus Associated With ACs

Hydrocephalus constitutes one of the main indications for surgical treatment of intracranial ACs. Hydrocephalus related to ACs may be due to flow obstruction or to faulty CSF reabsorption. Symptoms and signs of hydrocephalus in association with ACs do not substantially differ from those described for other causes of hydrocephalus (Table 13.2). Headaches, vomiting, and papilloedema constitute the standard symptoms of adult and older children hydrocephalus. In younger children, vomiting, drowsiness, decreased activity, increasing head circumference, split sutures, bulging fontanel, sun-setting eyes and squint, failure to thrive, and delayed development are frequent manifestations of hydrocephalus [6,16,20]. Macrocephaly, cranial asymmetry, and bulging of the adjacent bone may be found in large cysts in any location [6,16]. Headaches, cognitive deterioration, and dizziness/vertigo are usually regarded as characteristic of adult ACs with hydrocephalus. In patients with epilepsy, hydrocephalus may manifest with an increase in the number of seizures. Parinaud syndrome may occur in quadrigeminal cysts. A common presentation of suprasellar cysts and of cysts near the third ventricle is the "bobble-head doll" syndrome [6].

Notably, symptoms related to hydrocephalus usually predominate over those due to the AC. Often hydrocephalus evolves in a progressive manner or with features of "arrested hydrocephalus" [14]. In early reports, AC-related mortality was mainly due to undiagnosed hydrocephalus with catastrophic consequences [23].

TABLE 13.2   Clinical Presentation of ACs With or Without Associated Hydrocephalus

Symptom	Sign
Headaches / vomiting	Papilloedema / optic atrophy
Dizziness	6th CN palsy /squint
Seizures	Hemianopsia
Loss of vision / blurred vision / diplopia	Dysphasia
Loss of memory / behavioral symptoms / delayed psychomotor development	Hemiparesis / Long tract signs
Falls/ instability / syncope	Cranial asymmetry / Bulging of bone adjacent to cyst
Endocrine symptoms	

Infants: Macrocephaly / bulging fontanel / split sutures

Suprasellar and 3rd ventricle cysts:
Bobble-head doll syndrome

Quadrigeminal cysts:
Upward gaze palsy (Parinaud)

DIAGNOSIS OF AC-RELATED HYDROCEPHALUS

Initial reports on ACs generally included highly symptomatic cases or those with fully developed hydrocephalus. Many cases probably escaped detection due to the then available diagnostic tools, such as plain radiographs, tomography, ventriculography, pneumoencephalography, and cerebral angiography. All these techniques provided information about the site and relation of the lesion with the cisterns and ventricles. Angiography merely showed stretching and displacements of the cerebral arteries and veins by the space occupying lesion, although it ruled out the presence of tumors by the absence of pathological contrast staining.

At present, ultrasonography (US), CT, and MRI are the usual methods utilized in the evaluation of ACs and of associated hydrocephalus [6]. All these imaging methods depict the size and location of the cysts and supply information on the ventricular size and on the site of obstruction to CSF flow. Metrizamide-cisternography was utilized for demonstrating the communication of the cysts with the cisterns and subarachnoid space. Metrizamide-cisternography led to the classification of middle fossa ACs proposed by Galassi et al. [43]. Some new MRI sequences have replaced metrizamide-cisternography leading to the ceasing of its use.

MRI is useful for determining the ventricular size; it also shows the site of CSF obstruction, and the effects of the cysts on the surrounding brain. In addition, MRI can distinguish if the ventricular dilatation corresponds to active hydrocephalus or to brain atrophy. MRI shows the ventricles in the three planes of the space and is crucial for planning surgical approaches. MRI with special sequences (FIESTA) may also show the flow between compartments and permits assessing the success or failure of endoscopic procedures in ACs and hydrocephalus.

MRI studies allow the distinction of the diverse cystic lesions of the posterior fossa, such as trapped fourth ventricle, Dandy-Walker malformation and Dandy-Walker variant, Blake pouch, megacisterna magna, and ACs. MRI also contributes to the differential diagnosis against other cystic lesions (epidermoid, tumoral, parasitic). This technique is also utilized to monitor the pre- and postsurgical evolution of the cysts and that of the associated ventricular enlargement.

US studies are of upmost importance for the evaluation of AC-related pathologies in neonates and infants. US are cheap, innocuous, and easily available, which makes them the tool of election for children of this age. US can be used for the initial diagnosis, for monitoring the spontaneous evolution of both cyst and hydrocephalus, and also for assessing their response to treatments.

Antenatal US has greatly contributed to the assessment of the natural history of these cysts during the gestation. Pierre-Kahn et al. [41] performed a review of 54 fetuses in which prenatal US pointed to the presence of cystic lesions. In most cases, maternal MRI confirmed the diagnosis. In this study, the authors found a higher rate of supratentorial and interhemispheric cysts compared with only one case of a sylvian lesion. Pierre-Kahn et al. [41] also stressed the value of US for prenatal counseling and for deciding the most appropriate obstetric and neurosurgical conduct.

Di Rocco et al. [44] introduced prolonged *ICP monitoring* for deciding surgery in 11 children with sylvian ACs. This study showed normal ICP in Galassi type I cysts and increased ICP in Galassi type III cysts. This observation was not confirmed in the survey on middle fossa ACs performed by the same group, in which all patients studied with ICP monitoring showed normal values despite their Galassi type [30]. Helland and Wester performed *intracystic pressure* measurements in 38 patients during the surgeries for temporal ACs and found almost normal values in most cases. However, they found a significant correlation between intracystic pressure and level of preoperative complaints [45].

Some other diagnostic studies have also been used for detecting an eventual brain damage caused by the cysts. EEG, PET, and SPECT studies, and neurophysiological recording, showed variable results in regard to their utility for this purpose. Pre- and postoperative neuropsychological testing is increasingly utilized for indicating the need of surgical treatment and for assessing outcomes [8]. However, no single procedure has been shown to be capable of defining the actual degree of brain damage produced by the cyst. The diagnostic yield and usefulness of all the abovementioned ancillary diagnostic methods will be amply discussed in the corresponding chapters of this work.

MANAGEMENT OPTIONS FOR HYDROCEPHALUS IN ACs

There are three periods in the history of the management of ACs and of associated hydrocephalus:

1. Initially, the preferred approach consisted of the direct surgical attack to relieve the cyst pressure and to treat the associated hydrocephalus. These methods, although very effective, produced severe complications and had high mortality and morbidity rates.
2. The second period started with the extensive use of shunts, after which the preferred approach consisted of the placement of a cystoperitoneal (CP) shunt, a VP shunt, or a combination of both. Their use supposedly decreased procedural morbidity and mortality.
3. The third period commenced with the resurgence of endoscopic methods that reduced technical invasiveness and decreased long-term complications. Endoscopic procedures are increasingly utilized to overcome long-term effects of CSF drainage such as overshunting [46]. At present, neuroendoscopy has gained widespread favor and its indications in the management of AC and hydrocephalus are on the rise.

Ali et al. [47] analyzed 83 instances of ACs, and found no differences in outcomes among the surgical technique utilized (endoscopic fenestration, CP shunting, or craniotomy-based procedures). As expected, these three modalities of treatment continue to be used either in combination or sequentially. Apart from technical considerations, and even after the advent of advanced methods, the main concern consists on indicating which cysts should be operated. Patients with ACs are more likely to undergo surgery if they harbor large cysts, have hydrocephalus, or have experienced cyst rupture/hemorrhage [47]. On reviewing the current literature, it becomes obvious that there are no definite guidelines on the management of ACs and of the associated hydrocephalus. The decision to operate or not and the specific surgical technique have been traditionally based on the surgeon's preferences rather than on randomized

TABLE 13.3   Management Options for AC-Associated Hydrocephalus

Conservative treatment		
	Periodic, scheduled follow-up visits	
	Periodic imaging studies	
	As dictated by patients' clinical manifestation	

Surgical Treatments		
Temporary methods		External ventricular/cyst drainage Ventricular access device Free-hand puncture Stereotactic puncture
Permanent methods	Shunting procedures	Internal shunting (cysto-ventricular, cysto-subdural, cysto-cisterna magna shunting) Ventriculoperitoneal Cystoperitoneal Combined ventriculo-cystoperitoneal
	Open surgery (Craniotomy)	Craniotomy and cyst fenestration Combined with internal stents/shunts
	Endoscopic methods	Cysto-cisternostomy Cysto-ventriculostomy Endoscopic third ventriculostomy (isolated or associated)

studies or protocols [47]. A summary of management options is presented in Table 13.3.

Conservative Management

Previously, the mere presence of an AC in a neuroimaging study was regarded as a main indication for surgery. It was only after critically evaluating the outcomes and the complications derived from the surgery, especially those of CSF shunting, that many researchers started to recommend a more conservative attitude [6,8,11,46]. At present, most authors agree in advising observation only in: (1) patients with cysts that remain asymptomatic; (2) incidentally discovered cysts causing ventricular dilatation (not hydrocephalus); (3) patients with symptoms not directly related to the presence of the cyst or to ventriculomegaly. In a recent study of 488 children with intracranial ACs, observation only was indicated for 412 (84.43%) of cases [48].

The most important objection for a conservative attitude refers to instances of children in which the presence of hydrocephalus or of the cyst itself might be producing a latent neurological deterioration, e.g., those causing a negligible slowing of psychomotor development, or those producing mild cognitive or behavioral deterioration [8]. In any case, when a watch-and-see attitude is adopted, the neurosurgeon must perform periodic scheduled follow-up visits that include clinical and MRI assessment for a yet not determined period or at least until the age of 4 years. These scheduled follow-up visits can be changed as dictated by the patients' clinical evolution. In our view, there is no role for prophylactic surgery.

Surgical Management Options

Common surgical techniques include open surgery, endoscopic surgery, and CSF shunting procedures. Controversy still exists in regard to the optimal approach. The decision is influenced by the size and location of the cyst, coexisting hydrocephalus, proximity of important structures (nerves and vessels), and the surgeon's personal choice and experience [48]. Briefly, most authors agree in recommending surgery in patients with ACs that evolve with: (1) active hydrocephalus; (2) raised ICP; (3) unequivocal symptoms and signs of focal cerebral damage. Other authors support a not so strict attitude and prefer performing surgery aimed at preventing an eventual brain damage [45,49].

1. *Transient surgical measures.* Hydrocephalus in patients with ACs usually progresses slowly due to the following facts: (1) ICP in ACs usually does not exceed normal values; (2) the brain and the skull are capable of accommodating slow growing masses; and (3) progressive increases in CSF volume usually are compensated by displacements of blood and brain parenchyma. Accordingly, very rarely does hydrocephalus show up with life-threatening decompensation.
   In this event, acute hydrocephalus can be managed by an emergent external ventricular drainage as a temporary life-saving maneuver.
   In other situations, hydrocephalus can be transiently managed with a ventricular access device or with a free-hand or stereotactic cyst puncture.
2. *Definitive surgery.* Several options are normally utilized for permanent treatment of ACs and hydrocephalus: (1) open surgery with cyst excision or cyst fenestration; (2) endoscopic fenestration; (3) CSF drainage with VP or CP shunts; (4) various combinations of these techniques [6].
3. *Craniotomy.* Many authors favor craniotomy with open cyst fenestration for most cysts of all locations, especially with microsurgical techniques, as it carries a success rate of nearly 75% and has the advantage of avoiding the risks associated with shunting

[35,50]. In the European Cooperative Study, open surgery constituted the first-choice surgical option [50].

4. *Internal Shunting.* There exist several procedures for *internal shunting* of ACs [6]. Cysto-ventricular shunts allow the communication of the cyst with the ventricles and have the advantage of avoiding cyst overshunting. Quadrigeminal ACs can also be shunted internally to the cisterna magna. Cyst-subdural shunts have also been employed for internal cyst decompression [49], see Chapter 13, Surgical Techniques, Results, and Complications: Shunt Techniques— Cystosubdural Shunt, Cystoventricular Shunt/Stent, of Volume 2.

5. *Extracranial shunting.* Some authors favor the placement of *extracranial shunts,* such as VP or CP shunts, as the initial treatment of ACs and related hydrocephalus [23,26,32,51]. In cysts with ample communication with the subarachnoid space, VP alone may constitute the most effective treatment given that it may drain the ventricles and the cyst at the same time (Fig. 13.2). Evidently, a VP shunt in addition to cyst drainage becomes necessary in patients who develop hydrocephalus. Some authors recommend VP shunting as the initial procedure in small children with hydrocephalus or in those with "unspecific macrocephaly," especially in those younger than 2 years [16,32], see Chapter 12, Shunt Techniques—Cystoperitoneal Shunt, of Volume 2.

    The European Cooperative Study revealed that although only three centers preferred shunting procedures, 113 of 285 (39.6%) of cases were given a shunt [50]. Due to unsatisfactory clinical or imaging results, 78 (27.4%) patients required 113 additional surgeries. The need for a second surgical procedure was more frequent when cyst shunting was performed first [50].

    In addition to known problems of any CSF shunt, the major disadvantage of extracranial shunts consists of their propensity for developing overdrainage syndromes [46]. Many studies have confirmed this propensity for developing shunt dependence comprising "slit-cyst" syndrome, pseudotumor-like conditions, cranioencephalic disproportion, and acquired cerebellar tonsillar herniation [11,28,29,33]. Despite this drawback, approximately 50%– 65% of cases submitted to craniotomy later required some derivation of CSF for treatment of associated hydrocephalus or because of lack of improvement [23,35,52], see Chapter 14, Overdrainage Syndromes in Shunted Arachnoid Cysts, of Volume 2.

6. *Neuroendoscopic techniques.* The experience gained by neurosurgeons on endoscopic third ventriculostomy (ETV) in the management of hydrocephalus has favored the application of this method for the treatment of intracranial ACs. The technique is facilitated by the structure of the cyst with rather avascular walls and with a cavity that contains sufficient CSF to permit a good vision of its interior surface. In addition, the industry has developed new neuroendoscopy apparatuses that offer

safer and more refined management of AC-related hydrocephalus including HD cameras and better light source equipments. These features make ACs an ideal target for endoscopic fenestration. The main advances of neuroendoscopy consist of a miniaturization of the endoscopes and the design of a variety of new instruments that allow performing a minimally invasive technique, see Chapter 11, Endoscopic Techniques in Arachnoid Cyst Surgery, of Volume 2.

The precise localization of the planned targets can be improved with neuronavigation or with intraoperative US. Main disadvantages of the technique include the need for a dedicated specialized training and the difficulties arising from the identification of crucial anatomical structures (vessels and cranial nerves). Hopf and Perneczky [53] reported several variations of endoscopic procedures in 36 patients: endoscopic neurosurgery ($n = 14$), endoscopic assisted microneurosurgery ($n = 15$), and endoscopy controlled microneurosurgery ($n = 7$). Hydrocephalus was the main indication in 17 instances. The procedures were successful in 70% of the cases [53]. The best results were obtained in intraventricular and posterior fossa cysts and in those presenting with hydrocephalus and focal deficits [53].

Surgical Options According to AC Location

1. *Sylvian arachnoid cysts.* ACs of the middle cranial fossa account for approximately 50% of all intracranial cysts (Fig. 13.1A), 145 of 309 in the series reported by Al-Holou et al. [25]. The association of hydrocephalus with Sylvian ACs seems to be of rather rare occurrence. Tamburrini et al. [30] reported a survey of 45 pediatric neurosurgical services on the treatment of Sylvian ACs that demonstrated wide differences regarding management among the survey's responders. Di Rocco [7] also questioned the excessive tendency for operating middle fossa ACs.

   In a series of 40 patients with Sylvian ACs, six were given a VP shunt for hydrocephalus in addition to cyst fenestration, regardless which treatment had been performed first [20]. These authors also treated five of nine patients presenting with "unspecific macrocephaly" with a VP shunt [20]. In a series of children younger than 2 years of age, ventriculomegaly was found in only three of 22 instances of middle fossa ACs, although finally 18 of the whole group of 42 patients required CSF shunting and became shunt dependent over time [16].

   To avoid shunt complications, especially overshunting, many authors prefer using cyst fenestration by open or endoscopic surgery [16,23,28,34]. Sato et al. [11] also preferred craniotomy with cyst fenestration.

   We still use CP shunting in infants with sylvian cysts because open surgery seems to be more dangerous and neuroendoscopy is often useless in this age group, although we are progressively moving to using neuroendoscopy. In many instances we placed a combined ventriculo-cysto-peritoneal shunt with a Y connector to prevent differences of pressure between intracranial compartments. However, we no longer use valveless shunts and prefer using programmable valves instead.

Treatment of symptomatic temporal ACs was undertaken in 32 children with a purely endoscopic cysto-cisternostomy that led to improvement in 87.5% of cases and to an MRI reduction in cyst size in 71.9% of them, having few complications and a low recurrence rate [54].

2. *Posterior fossa ACs*. Posterior fossa ACs account for 15%−35% of all intracranial cysts (Figs. 13.3 and 13.4) and 38% (118 of 309 cysts) in the series of Al-Holou et al. [25]. Posterior fossa cysts produce hydrocephalus by blockage of the fourth ventricle in up to 90% of cases [3]. Another author documented that posterior fossa cysts produce hydrocephalus by a defective CSF reabsorption [14].

The treatment of lesions in this site should be based on the location and on the free communication of the cysts with the ventricles and/or cisterns. Accordingly, communicating cysts could be treated by ETV alone, ventriculocystostomy plus ETV, or by VP shunting. Another option consists of extracranial shunting of the ventricles and the posterior fossa cyst united by a three-way connector.

Some authors prefer using craniotomy with fenestration [3,14,36]. Samii et al. [55] documented a cohort of patients with posterior fossa ACs, the majority on the cerebellopontine angle, who were treated by a retrosigmoid approach. Sato et al. [11] treated their patients with posterior fossa cysts with several methods: craniotomy and excision ($n = 4$); craniotomy and subduroperitoneal shunt ($n = 1$); CP shunt ($n = 2$); and VP shunt ($n = 6$). Shim et al. [29] reported diverse treatment modalities in 18 posterior fossa cysts: endoscopic fenestration ($n = 3$); various shunt-related procedures ($n = 9$); and craniotomy with open fenestration ($n = 6$).

3. *Suprasellar and prepontine ACs*. Cysts arising from the suprasellar cisterns account for 5%−15% of all intracranial lesions. They are thought to originate from an anomalous development of the membrane of Liliequist. They usually grow upwards and occlude the foramina of Monro or anterior third ventricle producing obstructive hydrocephalus in up to 80% of instances [38] (Figs. 13.7−13.9). They produce a typical Mickey Mouse image in neuroimaging studies (Fig. 13.7).

Suprasellar ACs can be approached by open surgery using a pterional, subfrontal, or transventricular route. Anyway, some

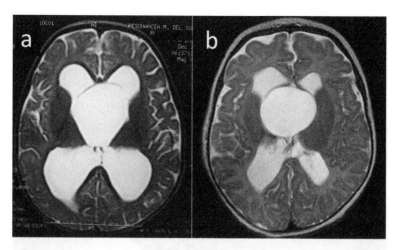

FIGURE 13.7 (A, B) MRI appearance of Mickey Mouse image in two instances of suprasellar cysts, causing bilateral hydrocephalus.

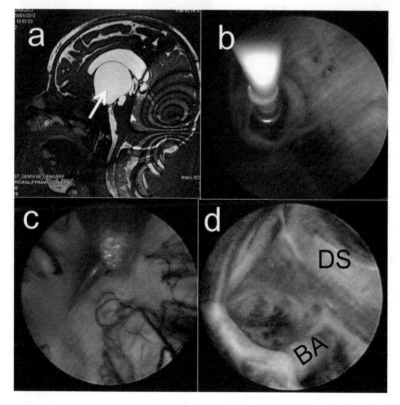

FIGURE 13.8 Suprasellar AC in a 4-month-old boy (A) FIESTA sequences showing the cyst (arrow); (B) endoscopic view of the cyst wall; (C) part of the cyst was extremely hard needing opening with scissors; (D) endoscopic view after ETV showing the dorsum sellae (DS) and the basilar artery (BA).

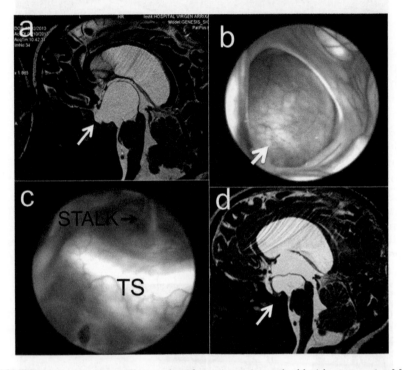

FIGURE 13.9   (A) Suprasellar arachnoid cyst in an 8-month-old girl preoperative MRI (FIESTA) view showing the cyst (arrow); (B) endoscopic view of the arachnoid cyst merging through a dilated foramen of Monro (arrow); (C) endoscopic view showing the pituitary stalk (PS) and dorsum sellae (DS); (D) postoperative MRI (FIESTA) showing decrease in size of the cyst (arrow).

suprasellar cysts do not resolve after craniotomy and require VP or CP derivation. Shunting alone by one of these two procedures seems to be inefficacious. Raimondi et al. [37] used a biventriculo-peritoneal shunt, followed by subfrontal craniotomy, partial cyst excision, and cysto-subarachnoid marsupialization.

Given their situation in the suprasellar cistern and their vicinity with the ventricular system, the preferred current approach for suprasellar cysts is with neuroendoscopy (Figs. 13. 8 and 13.9).

Wide endoscopic fenestration of the cyst walls allows the communication of the cyst with the ventricles (Fig. 13.9A–D). In addition, one can complete the procedure performing an ETV that resolves the accompanying hydrocephalus. This treatment was successful in five of seven cases reported by Hinojosa et al. [12]. With this combined approach (ventriculo-cysto-cisternostomy), the hydrocephalus and the mass effect of the cysts are satisfactorily resolved (Fig. 13.9D).

4. *Convexity ACs.* ACs situated at the cerebral convexity represent 12%–17% of all intracranial cysts (Fig. 13.1B). In Zada et al.'s [16] experience there were five (12%) convexity cysts, and only one presented with hydrocephalus. This feature attests that hydrocephalus is rarely present in convexity lesions. In a series of 309 ACs, only 12 were situated at the convexities [25]. Small lesions are usually asymptomatic and rarely require treatment. CP shunting was used in eight (13%) convexity cysts in a study of 46 ACs [51]. However, large cysts may produce symptoms by their mass effect and then they need treatment that is best performed by a craniotomy or by endoscopic fenestration centered on the cyst.

5. *Quadrigeminal region ACs.* Cysts arising from the quadrigeminal plate region account for 5%–10% of all intracranial ACs (Fig. 13.10). In the surgical series of Ersahin et al. [56], all patients ($n = 17$) presented

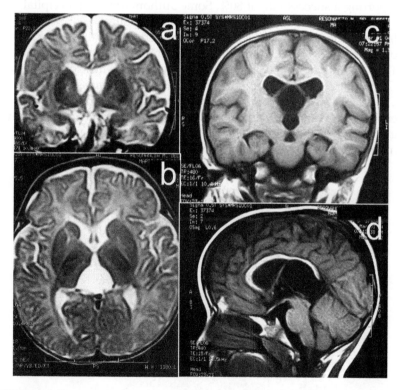

FIGURE 13.10 MRI images corresponding to a 1-year-old boy with a quadrigeminal arachnoid cyst (A) coronal view showing marked pericerebral collections and widened sulci; (B) axial cuts; (C) coronal view showing resolution of the pericerebral collections of fluid at age 3 years; (D) sagittal MRI showing the unchanged cyst size and absence of hydrocephalus.

III. PREVALENCE AND NATURAL HISTORY OF ARACHNOID CYSTS

with hydrocephalus and were treated with endoscopic fenestration plus ETV. This procedure was successful in nine children, but five of eight patients later required a VP shunt [56]. Cinalli et al. [39] reported a success rate of 78% of their 14 cases submitted to endoscopic treatment and of 90% when endoscopy was used as first procedure. The best results were obtained by combining endoscopic cystoventriculostomy with ETV [39].

6. *Intraventricular ACs.* ACs originating within the ventricles account for approximately 5% of all intracranial cysts (Fig. 13.11). In 1992, we reported three instances of hydrocephalus and lateral ventricle cysts that were treated: one by craniotomy and cyst excision and the other two by CP shunting; in one of them endoscopy was used for cyst fenestration [18]. Intraventricular ACs often present with hydrocephalus. Tamburrini et al. [57] documented hydrocephalus in 15 of 26 ventricular cysts, which were treated with neuroendoscopy reporting a success rate of 80%. Some authors utilize an occipital approach for performing the cystoventriculostomy.

7. *Intraparenchymal ACs.* ACs rarely are located within the cerebral parenchyma without communication with the subarachnoid space. They are rather situated in the proximity of the ventricles. El-Ghandour et al. [40] have reported them as a separate subgroup. Their 12 pediatric patients with these cysts were submitted to endoscopic cystoventriculostomy and three (25%) were additionally given an ETV for hydrocephalus. There was a significant improvement in 10 (83.3%) patients [40].

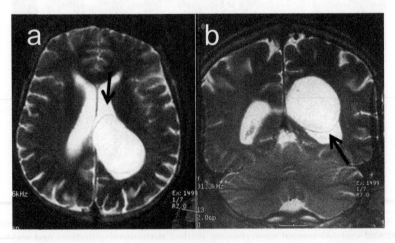

FIGURE 13.11   MRI of a 16-year-old girl with severe positional headaches diagnosed with a left lateral ventricle arachnoid cyst before ventriculocystostomy, MRI (A) in axial cut, and (B) in coronal view (arrows).

8. *Cerebellar tonsil herniation and posterior fossa ACs.* The association of posterior fossa ACs with tonsillar descent and syringomyelia has been documented exceptionally [23,25,26,48]. Plugging of the foramen magnum by the cyst itself can produce hydrocephalus and syringomyelia by obstructing the CSF flow [26]. A different mechanism attributes the development of hydrocephalus, acquired Chiari, and syringomyelia to the displacement of the cerebellar tonsils within the foramen magnum primarily caused by the push on the tonsils by a retrocerebellar AC [27]. In a recent revision from our institution the association of tonsillar descent and posterior fossa ACs emerged as a condition more frequent than was anteriorly thought [13]. These authors reported the association of posterior fossa AC-tonsillar descent in 10 patients. Six patients had, in addition, a cervical or cervicothoracic syrinx. Suboccipital decompression was performed in 6 of the10 patients. Three of 10 individuals with hydrocephalus were treated: one with a VP shunt and two with an ETV [13]. These authors recommend that hydrocephalus should be properly addressed before treating the AC. In our view, this association should be treated by ETV first followed by posterior fossa decompression if required.

OUTCOME

The goals of surgical treatment for ACs consist of the relief of patients' clinical symptoms associated to the cyst mass effect and eventually of those related to hydrocephalus. The reported mortality rate in earlier reports was as high as 8% [58] and has practically disappeared in modern series. Talamonti et al. [5] documented that 40 of 44 (91%) of their symptomatic patients who were treated by neuroendoscopy were clinically much improved, 9% were unchanged, and none worsened. Neuroimaging outcomes often document little or no decrease in the cysts' size but increasing experience on this pathology has demonstrated that cyst reduction does not parallel clinical results [49]. In a revision of ACs in 156 adults, 82% of patients became asymptomatic or had insignificant symptoms, 12% showed no improvement, and 6% had worsened [49]. Regarding 48 pediatric cases, 82% were much improved, 14% reported no improvement, and 4% were worsened [59].

The outcome of hydrocephalus in ACs does not differ from the reported results for hydrocephalus pertaining to other etiologies. In this regard, most patients usually fully recover following any option that addresses appropriately the hydrocephalus. The final outcome of patients with ventricular dilatation in the context of ACs is mainly related to the location and size of the underlying cyst and to the success of the modality of treatment used.

CONCLUSIONS

Hydrocephalus constitutes an often-found associated condition in patients with intracranial ACs. It is usually due to blockage of the CSF pathways by the cyst. An attractive theory supports the view that the development of the AC itself is motivated by a latent derangement in CSF dynamics and that the cyst constitutes a localized form of hydrocephalus. This reasoning indicates that clinical manifestations do not resolve with treatments that address only the local mass effect of the cyst. Symptoms and signs of AC-related hydrocephalus do not substantially differ from those that occur in hydrocephalus of other causes. There are three main approaches in the treatment of this condition: those based on cyst communication with the subarachnoid spaces, those based on the derivation of CSF, and those that utilize neuroendoscopic methods. At present, there are no agreed guidelines in the decision-making of these combined pathologies. Given the collateral effects of shunting procedures, neuroendoscopic treatments are emerging as the treatment of choice. The ideal option consists of the method that offers the highest success rate using a single procedure for treating the hydrocephalus and the AC at the same time.

References

[1] Robinson RG. Intracranial collections of fluid with local bulging of the skull. J Neurosurg 1955;12:345−53.
[2] Gruszkiewicz J, Peyser E. Supratentorial arachnoid cyst associated with hydrocephalus. J Neurol Neurosurg Psychiatry 1965;28:438−41.
[3] Harrison MJG. Cerebral arachnoid cysts in children. J Neurol Neurosurg Psychiatry 1971;34:316−23.
[4] Martínez-Lage JF, Poza M, López F. Arachnoid cyst as a complication of ventricular shunting. Childs Nerv Syst 1991;7:356−7.
[5] Talamonti G, D'Aliberti G, Picano M, Debernardi A, Collice M. Intracranial cysts containing cerebrospinal fluid-like fluid: results of endoscopic neurosurgery in a series of 64 consecutive cases. Neurosurgery 2011;68:788−803.
[6] Wilkinson CC, Winston KR. Congenital arachnoid cysts and Dandy-Walker complex. In: Albright AL, Pollack IF, Adelson PD, editors. Principles and practice of pediatric neurosurgery. 2nd ed. New York, Stuttgart: Thieme; 2008. p. 162−86.
[7] Di Rocco C. Sylvian fissure arachnoid cysts: we do operate on them but should we? (Commentary). Childs Nerv Syst 2010;26:173−5.
[8] Lee JY, Kim JW, Phi JH, Kim SK, Cho BK, Wang KC. Enlarging arachnoid cysts: a false alarm for infants. Childs Nerv Syst 2012;28:1203−11.
[9] Martínez-Lage JF, Ruíz-Maciá D, Valentí JA, Poza M. Development of a middle fossa arachnoid cyst: a theory on its pathogenesis. Childs Nerv Syst 1999;15:94−7.

[10] Gosalakkal J. Intracranial arachnoid cysts in children: a review of pathogenesis, clinical features, and management. Pediatr Neurol 2002;26:93–8.

[11] Sato H, Sato N, Katayama S, Tamaki N, Matsumoto S. Effective shunt-independent treatment for primary middle fossa arachnoid cyst. Childs Nerv Syst 1991;7:375–81.

[12] Hinojosa J, Esparza J, Muñoz MJ, Valencia J. Tratamiento endoscópico de los quistes aracnoideos supraselares. Neurocirugia (Astur) 2001;12:482–8.

[13] Galarza M, López López-Guerrero A, Martínez-Lage JF. Posterior fossa arachnoid cysts and cerebellar tonsillar descent: short review. Neurosurg Rev 2010;33:305–14.

[14] Di Rocco C, Di Trapani G, Iannelli A. Arachnoid cysts of the fourth ventricle and "arrested" hydrocephalus. Surg Neurol 1979;42:467–71.

[15] Pattisapu JV, Olavarria G, Gregg CA. Arachnoid cysts: a diffuse spinal fluid absorption abnormality. Cerebrosp Fluid Res 2009;6(Suppl 1):530.

[16] Zada G, Krieger MD, McNatt SA, Bowen I, McComb JG. Pathogenesis and treatment of intracranial arachnoid cysts in pediatric patients younger than 2 years of age. Neurosurg Focus 2007;22(2):E1.

[17] Kim TG, Kim DS, Choi JU. Are arachnoid cysts localized hydrocephali? Pediatr Neurosurg 2010;46:362–7.

[18] Martínez-Lage JF, Pérez-Espejo MA, Almagro MJ, López López-Guerrero A. Hydrocephalus and arachnoid cysts. Childs Nerv Syst 2011;27:1643–52.

[19] Mattei TA, Bond BJ, Sambhara D, Goulart CR, Lin JJ. Benign extracerebral fluid collection in infancy as a risk factor for the development of de novo intracranial arachnoid cysts. J Neurosurg Pediatr 2013;12:555–64.

[20] Levy ML, Meltzer HS, Hughes S, Aryan HE, Yoo K, Amar AP. Hydrocephalus in children with middle fossa arachnoid cysts. J Neurosurg 2004;101(Suppl 2):25–31.

[21] Martínez-Lage JF, Poza M, Rodriguez Costa T. Bilateral temporal arachnoid cysts in neurofibromatosis. J Child Neurol 1993;8:383–5.

[22] Martínez-Lage JF, Casas C, Fernández MA, Puche A, Rodríguez Costa T, Poza M. Macrocephaly, dystonia, and bilateral temporal arachnoid cysts: glutaric aciduria type 1. Childs Nerv Syst 1994;10:198–203.

[23] Pascual-Castroviejo I, Roche MC, Bermejo AM, Arcas J, Blazquez MG. Primary intracranial arachnoid cysts: a study of 67 childhood cases. Childs Nerv Syst 1991;7:257–63.

[24] Schievink WI, Huston III J, Torres VE, Marsh WR. Intracranial cysts in autosomal dominant polycystic kidney disease. J Neurosurg 1995;83:1004–7.

[25] Al-Holou WN, Yew AY, Boomsaad ZE, Garton HJL, Muraszko KM, Maher CO. Prevalence and natural history of arachnoid cysts in children. J Neurosurg Pediatr 2010;5:578–85.

[26] Toki T, Okamoto S, Yamagata S, Konishi T. Syringomyelia associated with a posterior fossa arachnoid cyst. Illustration of two cases. J Neurosurg 1997;86:907.

[27] Martínez-Lage JF, Almagro MJ, Ros de San Pedro J, Ruíz-Espejo A, Felipe-Murcia M. Regression of syringomyelia and tonsillar herniation after posterior fossa arachnoid cyst excision. Case report and literature review. Neurocirugia (Astur) 2007;18:227–31.

[28] Rabiei K, Högfeldt MJ, Doria-Medina R, Tisell M. Surgery for intracranial arachnoid cysts in children—a prospective long-term study. Childs Nerv Syst 2016;32:1257–63.

[29] Shim KW, Lee YH, Park EK, Park YS, Choi JU, Kim DS. Treatment options for arachnoid cysts. Childs Nerv Syst 2009;25:1459–66.

[30] Tamburrini G, Del Fabbro MD, Di Rocco C. Sylvian fissure arachnoid cysts: a survey on their diagnostic work-out and practical management. Childs Nerv Syst 2008;24:593–604.

[31] Steiger HJ. Preventive neurosurgery: population-wide check-up examinations and correction of asymptomatic pathologies of the nervous system. Acta Neurochir (Wien) 2006;148:1075–83.

[32] Marinov M, Undjian S, Wetzka P. An evaluation of the surgical treatment of intracranial arachnoid cysts in children. (1989). Childs Nerv Syst 1989;5:177–83.

[33] Sommer IEC, Smit LME. Congenital supratentorial arachnoidal and giant cysts in children: a clinical study with arguments for a conservative approach. Childs Nerv Syst 1997;13:8–12.
[34] Galarza M, Pomata HB, Pueyrredón F, Bartuluchi M, Zuccaro GN, Monges JA. Symptomatic supratentorial arachnoid cysts in children. Pediatr Neurol 2002;27: 180–5.
[35] Fewell ME, Levy ML, Mc Comb JG. Surgical treatment of 95 children with 102 intracranial arachnoid cysts. Pediatr Neurosurg 1996;25:167–73.
[36] Galassi E, Tognetti F, Frank F, Faglioli L, Nasi MT, Gaist G. Infratentorial arachnoid cysts. J Neurosurg 1985;63:210–17.
[37] Raimondi AJ, Shimoji T, Gutierrez FA. Suprasellar cysts: surgical treatment and results. Childs Brain 1980;7:57–72.
[38] Pierre-Kahn A, Capelle L, Braune R, Saint-Rose C, Renier D, Rappaport R, et al. Presentation and management of suprasellar arachnoid cysts: review of 20 cases. J Neurosurg 1990;73:355–9.
[39] Cinalli G, Spennato P, Columbano L, Ruggiero C, Aliberti F, Trischitta V, et al. Neuroendoscopic treatment of arachnoid cysts of the quadrigeminal cistern: a series of 14 cases. J Neurosurg Pediatr 2010;6:489–97.
[40] El-Ghandour NMF. Endoscopic treatment of intraparenchymal arachnoid cysts in children. J Neurosurg Pediatr 2014;14:501–7.
[41] Pierre-Kahn A, Hanlo P, Sonigo P, Parisot D, McConell RS. The contribution of prenatal diagnosis to the understanding of malformative intracranial cysts: state of the art. Childs Nerv Syst 2000;16:618–26.
[42] Mattei TA. Pediatric arachnoid cysts and subdural hygromas in early infancy: challenging the direction of the causality paradigm (Letter). Neurosurgery 2014;74: E150–3.
[43] Galassi E, Tognetti F, Gaist G, Faglioli L, Frank F, Frank G. CT scan and metrizamide cisternography in arachnoid cysts of the middle cranial fossa: classification and pathophysiological aspects. Surg Neurol 1982;17:363–9.
[44] Di Rocco C, Tamburrini G, Caldarelli M, Velardi F, Santini P. Prolonged ICP monitoring in sylvian arachnoid cysts. Surg Neurol 2003;60:211–18.
[45] Helland CA, Wester K. Intracystic pressure in patients with temporal arachnoid cysts: a prospective study of preoperative complaints and postoperative outcome. J Neurol Neurosurg Psychiatry 2007;78:620–3.
[46] Martínez-Lage JF, Ruíz-Espejo AM, Almagro MJ, Alfaro R, Felipe-Murcia M, López López-Guerrero A. CSF overdrainage in shunted intracranial arachnoid cysts: a series and review. Childs Nerv Syst 2009;25:1061–9.
[47] Ali M, Bennardo M, Almenawer SA, Zagzoog N, Smith AA, Dao D, et al. Exploring predictors of surgery and comparing operative treatment approaches for pediatric intracranial arachnoid cysts: a case series of 83 patients. J Neurosurg Pediatr 2015;16: 275–82.
[48] Huang JH, Mei WZ, Chen Y, Chen JW, Lin ZX. Analysis of clinical characteristics of intracranial arachnoid cysts in 488 pediatric cases. Int J Exp Med 2015;8:18343–50.
[49] Helland CA, Wester K. A population-based study of intracranial arachnoid cysts: clinical and neuroimaging outcomes following surgical cyst decompression in adults. J Neurol Neurosurg Psychiatry 2007;78:1129–35.
[50] Oberbauer RW, Haase J, Pucher R. Arachnoid cysts in children: a European cooperative study. Childs Nerv Syst 1992;8:281–6.
[51] Zhang B, Zhang Y, Ma Z. Long-term results of cystoperitoneal shunt placement for the treatment of arachnoid cysts in children. J Neurosurg Pediatr 2012;10:302–5.
[52] Gelabert-Gonzalez M. Quistes aracnoideos intracraneales. Rev Neurol 2004;39: 1161–6.

[53] Hopf N, Perneczky A. Endoscopic neurosurgery and endoscope-assisted microneuro-surgery for the treatment of intracranial cysts. Neurosurgery 1998;43:13301337.

[54] El-Ghandour NM. Endoscopic treatment of middle cranial fossa arachnoid cysts in children. J Neurosurg Pediatr 2012;9:231—8.

[55] Samii M, Carvalho GA, Schuhmann MU. Arachnoid cysts of the posterior fossa. Surg Neurol 1999;51:376—82.

[56] Ersahin Y, Kesikçi H. Endoscopic management of quadrigeminal arachnoid cysts. Childs Nerv Syst 2009;25:569—76.

[57] Tamburrini G, D'Angelo L, Paternoster G, Massimi L, Caldarelli M, Di Rocco C. Endoscopic management of intra and paraventricular CSF cysts. Childs Nerv Syst 2007;23:645—51.

[58] Richard KE, Dahl K, Sanker P. Long-term follow-up of children and juveniles with arachnoid cysts. Childs Nerv Syst 1989;5:184—7.

[59] Helland CA, Wester K. A population-based study of intracranial arachnoid cysts: clinical and neuroimaging outcomes following surgical cyst decompression in children. J Neurosurg 2006;105(5Suppl):385—90.

Further Reading

Bright R. Report of medical cases selected with a view of illustrating symptoms and cure of diseases by reference to morbid anatomy. Diseases of the brain and nervous system, vol. II. London: Longman; 1831. p. 437—9.

Choi TG, Kim DS, Choi JU. Are arachnoid cysts localized hydrocephali? Pediatr Neurosurg 2010;46:362—7.

Cinalli G, Peretta P, Spennato P, Savarese L, Varone A, Vedova P, et al. Neuroendoscopic management of interhemispheric cysts in children. J Neurosurg 2006;105(Suppl 3): 192—202.

García Santos JM, Martínez-Lage J, Gilabert Ubeda A, Capel Alemán A, Climent Oltrá V. Arachnoid cysts of the middle cranial fossa: a consideration on their origins based on imaging. Neuroradiology 1993;35:355—8.

Lewis AJ. Infantile hydrocephalus caused by arachnoid cyst, case report. J Neurosurg 1962;19:431—4.

Martínez-Lage JF, Poza M, Sola J, Puche A. Congenital arachnoid cyst of the lateral ventricles in children. Childs Nerv Syst 1992;8:203—6.

Quain R. Large cyst from the cavity of the arachnoid. Trans Pathol Soc 1855;6:8—10.

Santamarta D, Aguas J, Ferrer E. The natural history of arachnoid cysts: endoscopic and cine-mode MRI evidence of a slit-valve mechanism. Min Inv Neurosurg 1995;38:133—7.

PART IV

NEUROIMAGING

14

Radiological Workup, CT, MRI

Johan Wikström

Uppsala University Hospital, Uppsala, Sweden

Arachnoid Cysts: Epidemiology, Biology, and Neuroimaging
DOI: http://dx.doi.org/10.1016/B978-0-12-809932-2.00014-4

RECOMMENDATIONS—LEVEL OF EVIDENCE

Level I

There is no Level I evidence available regarding the radiological workup of arachnoid cyst (AC).

Level II

The delineation of ACs can be assessed with high accuracy with computed tomography (CT) cisternography after intrathecal iodine contrast agent administration, but also with noninvasive MR cisternography.

The communication between ACs and surrounding subarachnoid space can be assessed with high accuracy with CT cisternography after intrathecal iodine contrast agent administration, but also with noninvasive flow-sensitive magnetic resonance imaging (MRI) techniques.

Diffusion weighted MRI is a highly accurate technique for differentiation between an AC and an epidermoid.

INTRODUCTION

Radiology has an important role in several steps in the workup of ACs. It aids detection, delineation, differential diagnosis, presurgical evaluation and follow-up after treatment. The techniques that are used for these purposes are CT and MRI.

IMAGING TECHNIQUES

Computed Tomography

In CT, differences in electron density cause different X-ray attenuation and hence differences in image gray scale. Modern CT scanners acquire contiguous slices of very thin thickness which enables reconstruction of images in any desired plane. Soft tissue contrast in CT is considerably lower than in MRI and it has the further disadvantage of ionizing radiation, which is a concern especially in the pediatric population. Advantages include that it is more widely available and cheaper, which makes it often used for initial detection.

Magnetic Resonance Imaging

MRI is the most important imaging technique for the further assessment of ACs. MRI does not involve the use of ionizing radiation, has the advantage of superior soft tissue contrast and also the possibility for tissue characterization by means of complementary information from different types of sequences. Image contrast depends to a large degree from tissue concentration of free water. Depending on sequence type, contrast can however also be affected by, e.g., content of fat, hemorrhage, calcium, iron, or other metals with magnetic properties, which permit improved lesion characterization compared with CT. The two main MR sequence types are T1- and T2-weighted; where T1 and T2 denotes relaxatation times, i.e., how fast the tissue magnetization regains the original state after being subjected to a radiowave. T2-weighted images are the most important for detection of pathology, with increasing signal intensity with increase in water content. In T1-weighted images, the contrast is more or less the opposite, with low signal intensity from fluid. In T1-weighted images, high signal intensity is mainly seen in fat, some blood products, and calcium compounds but also in contrast agent enhancing lesions. MRI enables not only morphological imaging but also the aqcuisition of different types of functional information. MR sequences can for instance be made sensitive to flow. In a T2-weighted spin echo sequence without flow compensation, flow in blood vessels and CSF spaces will cause signal loss, and with the so-called phase contrast MR technique it is possible to detect and quantify flow and flow velocity (Fig. 14.1) [1].

Cisternography

For detailed assessment of lesions in the subarachnoid space; there are different types of contrast agent-based cisternography techniques, using CT, MRI, or radionuclide techniques[2–4]. Common to all three is the injection of a contrast agent (ioidine, gadolinium, or radionuclide) into the intrathecal space by lumbar puncture. Of these three, CT is the most used. In this technique, CT of the head is performed after intrathecal administration of an iodine contrast agent, with the head lowered. If imaging is performed shortly after contrast agent administration, it will be possible to outline noncommunicating ACs. Contrast agent-based MR cisternography is seldom used, since the intrathecal injection of the gadolinium-based contrast agents used for MRI is not universally accepted as safe, and especially so after recent reports of gadolinium deposition in different organs including the brain [5]. Radionuclide-based cisternography is an outdated technique, being both much less available and having poorer spatial resolution than CT.

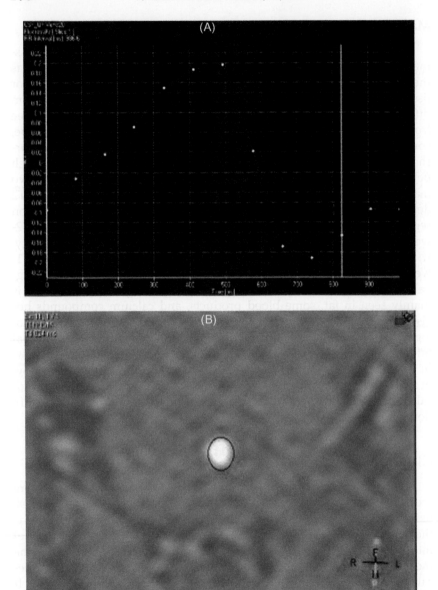

FIGURE 14.1 Images from phase contrast MRI sequence. Flow velocity curve in cerebral aqueduct at different time points of the cardiac cycle (A), and image showing placement of region-of-interest (B).

DETECTION

Although ACs may be symptomatic, they are often incidental findings made at MR or CT examinations performed because of symptoms not related to the cyst. They are detected from the finding of a localized widening of the subarachnoid space, which can be made about as easy with CT as with MRI. Common localizations include the middle cranial fossa and the retrocerebellar space, but they can be localized anywhere at the cerebral and cerebellar margins [6], in the spinal subarachnoid space [7,8], and infrequently also intraventricularly [9]. Examples of ACs in different locations are given in Fig. 14.2. Depending on their size, they may cause compression and deformation of the adjacent brain parenchyma. The cyst wall is very thin compared with the resolution of both CT and MRI and is often difficult to detect on routine images. For delineation of soft tissue structures within fluid, e.g., nerves, vessels but also cyst walls, highly T2-weighted MR sequences with high spatial resolution have been developed [10]. A finding that supports the diagnosis of an AC is a local thinning of the adjacent skull bone (Fig. 14.2C). Since ACs are typically of developmental origin, they may be detected early in life, and sometimes even intrauterine, by ultrasound or MRI [11] (Fig. 14.3), see Chapter 15, Arachnoid Cyst—Prenatal Detection, Management, and Perinatal Outcome.

DIFFERENTIAL DIAGNOSIS

ACs must be differentiated from other cystic lesions within the intracranial and intraspinal compartments. Depending on location, these differential diagnoses include mega cisterna magna, neurenteric cysts, porencephalic cysts, colloid cysts, ependymal cysts, choroid plexus cysts, cystic tumors, cystic infectious lesions, and subdural hematomas [12].

Examples of differential diagnoses are given in Fig. 14.4. In the posterior fossa, a retrocerebellar fluid collection could represent either an AC or an enlarged cisterna magna (mega cisterna magna), which is a very common pitfall in the diagnosis of a retrocerebellar AC, particularly if the diagnosis is performed by neurosurgeons. Absence of compression of the cerebellum and free communication with the surrounding subarachnoid space speaks for a mega cisterna magna rather than an AC (Fig. 14.4A–C). When in doubt, a CT cisternography with lumbar contrast instillation and an immediate CT scan with the patient lying on the back will be decisive. In a mega cisterna there will be an immediate contrast filling of the fluid compartment.

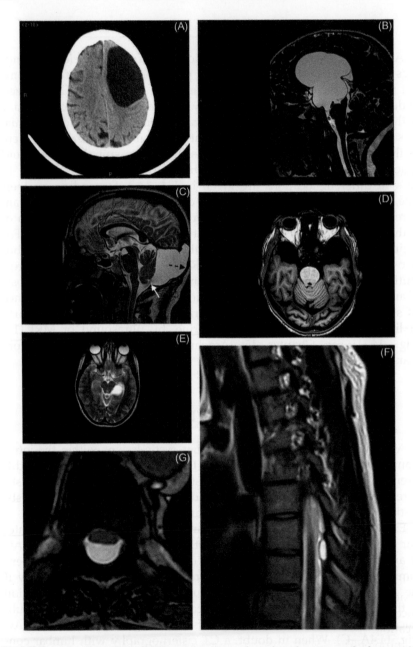

FIGURE 14.2 Examples of different locations of arachnoid cysts: cerebral convexity (A), suprasellar (B), retrocerebellar (C), bilateral middle fossa (D), ambient cistern (E), spinal extradural (F), and spinal intradural (G).

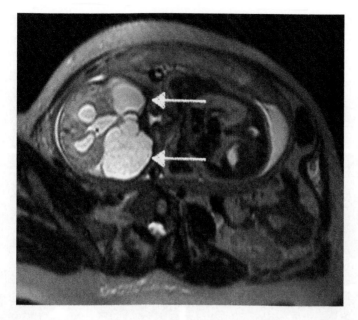

FIGURE 14.3   Fetal MRI showing hydrocephalus and bilateral temporal arachnoid cysts (arrows).

One further important differential diagnosis for an AC is an epidermoid. Epidermoids are developmental cystic lesions. They are most often found in the suprasellar cistern or cerebellopontine angle, but can be located anywhere in the subarachnoid space, also in the spinal canal, and rarely also in the brain parenchyma and bone. At CT, epidermoids appear to be often quite similar to ACs, with attenuation similar to cerebrospinal fluid. The distinction can on the other hand almost always be made easy with MRI, where the most useful sequence for this purpose is the diffusion weighted sequence, on which epidermoids show very high signal because of diffusion restriction (Fig. 14.4D); whereas ACs have unrestricted diffusion and low signal [13] (Fig. 14.4E).

A porencephalic cyst is a cystic lesion within the brain parenchyma, following an event with tissue destruction, e.g., vascular, traumatic, toxic, or infectious. It has identical attenuation and MRI signal appearance as an AC, but can be differentiated from the latter based on location.

Intraventricular ACs are very rare [9]. Other intraventricular cystic lesions include colloid cysts, subependymal cysts, and choroid plexus cysts. A colloid cyst is most often located at the foramen of Monro, and has usually characteristic high CT attenuation. Ependymal cysts have identical attenuation and MRI signal appearance as ACs, and cannot be

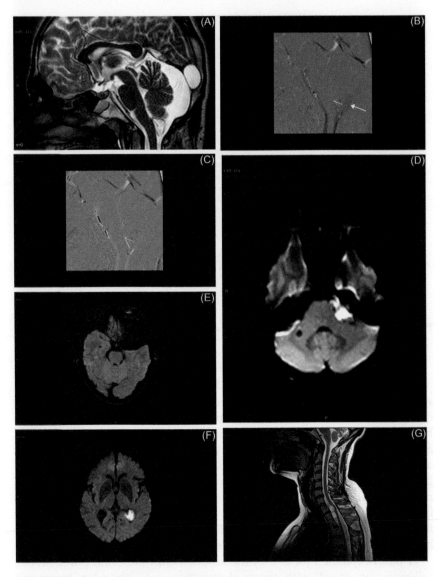

FIGURE 14.4   Examples of differential diagnoses for arachnoid cysts. A retrocerebellar fluid collection may represent an arachnoid cyst or an enlarged cisterna magna (mega cisterna magna) (A). In this case, phase contrast MRI (two time points in B–C) reveals free flow into the fluid (arrow in (B)) which supports a diagnosis of a mega cisterna magna. Diffusion weighted MR images of epidermoid (D) with hindered diffusion causing high signal intensity, and arachnoid cyst (E) with unhindered diffusion causing low signal intensity. Diffusion weighted MRI of choroid plexus cyst in the left lateral ventricle (F). There is high signal because of intracystic material (e.g., inflammatory cells and cholesterol clefts) causing hindered diffusion. Sagittal T2-weighted MRI of patient with neurenteric cyst (G). There is a bilocular cystic lesion in the anterior spinal intradural compartment and associated vertebral anomalies.

reliably differentiated by imaging. Cystic lesions of the choroid plexus are differentiated from ACs/ependymal cysts by their location, the expansion of the choroid plexus as opposed to ACs that will cause choroid plexus compression, and also by their often low diffusion (Fig. 14.4F).

A rare differential diagnosis anterior to the brainstem and spinal cord is the neurenteric cyst. A neurenteric cyst is believed to be the result of an incomplete separation between the notochord and the foregut. It includes a cystic lesion anterior to the neural axis, commonly associated with vertebral body malformations (Fig. 14.4G) and sometimes a visible connection between the subarachnoid space and the alimentary tract [14].

Tumors in the subarachnoid space include meningiomas, schwannomas, and metastases. Most often, these are easy to distinguish from ACs based on their solid components. Rarely, for instance, meningiomas may be almost purely cystic. In these cases imaging after i.v. contrast medium administration can differentiate the two, where an enhancing capsule is typical in meningiomas but not in ACs. Similarly, some infectious lesions are cystic, e.g., hydatid cysts and neurocysticercosis; and may resemble ACs [12].

Chronic subdural hematomas may have similar CT attenuation as ACs, whereas at MRI, the signal pattern is never completely identical. One problem may be to differentiate a subdural hematoma from an AC with hemorrhage. The obvious clue to a correct diagnosis is the different locations; i.e., the subarachnoid versus the subdural space.

DELINEATION

An AC can often be reasonably well delineated by both CT and MRI. The wall, however, is seldom seen on CT without contrast administration, and not always on routine MRI sequences either. For precise delineation CT cisternography may be performed. Nowadays, heavily T2-weighted MRI sequences with thin slices and high in-plane spatial resolution have increased the ability to noninvasively delineate these lesions considerably [10] (Fig. 14.2B).

PRETREATMENT EVALUATION

Different imaging parameters are reviewed before choosing between conservative or surgical treatment. These include the degree of compression of nearby structures, presence of CSF circulation obstruction,

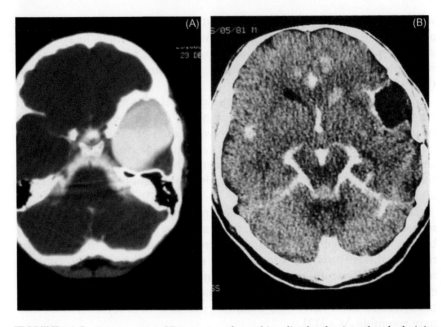

FIGURE 14.5   Postoperative CT images performed imediately after intrathecal administration of iodine contrast medium, with the head lowered (CT cisternography), in two
patients with left temporal arachnoid cysts. In (A), there is obvious presence of contrast
medium within the left temporal arachnoid cyst which confirms communication with the
surrounding subarachnoid space. In (B), there is no opacification of the left temporal cyst,
and hence no proven communication. *Source: Images courtesy of Prof. Knut Wester.*

and edema. All of these may be assessed by CT but more reliably so
with MRI. An assessment of any communication between the cyst and
the surrounding subarachnoid space is also of vital importance in
the decision-making. CT cisternography can give this information
(Fig. 14.5), but also flow-sensitive MRI sequences (T2-weighted spin
echo without flow compensation or phase contrast MRI) [15] (Figs. 14.1,
14.2C, 14.4A–C).

EVALUATION AFTER SURGERY

In the immediate postsurgical period, radiology can assist by detection of complications such as bleeding, infarction, or hydrocephalus.
Ischemic lesions may be detected by CT, but may be missed in the
hyperacute period. Diffusion weighted MRI on the other hand is a very
sensitive technique for this evaluation [16]. Acute hemorrhage can be
detected confidently with both CT and MRI [16]. For detection of rem-
nants after previous hemorrhage, which may be a cause of scarring and

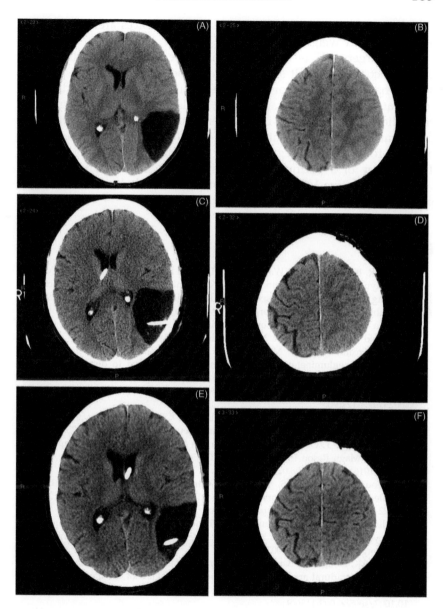

FIGURE 14.6 CT images of left convexity aracnoid cyst before (A−B) and at two time points after shunt treatment (C−D and E−F). After shunt placement, there is progressive decrease in cyst size, ventricle compression, and sulcal effacement.

CSF flow obstruction, blood sensitive MRI sequences are needed, such as susceptibility weighted imaging [17].

After surgery, CT or MRI can verify a decrease in cyst size and in mass effect (Fig. 14.6). It should however be appreciated that previous studies have shown no correlation between neuroimaging and clinical results after AC surgery in adults [18], while a corresponding significant correlation was observed in children, but only when results were dichotomized [19]. In the later follow-up after surgery, the role of radiology is to detect cyst regrowth and to evaluate fenestration patency. The patency of a performed cyst fenestration is most often assessed with flow-sensitive MRI techniques, or, alternatively by CT cisternography, analogous to the workup before treatment.

References

[1] Nitz WR, Bradley Jr. WG, Watanabe AS, Lee RR, Burgoyne B, O'Sullivan RM, et al. Flow dynamics of cerebrospinal fluid: assessment with phase-contrast velocity MR imaging performed with retrospective cardiac gating. Radiology 1992;183(2):395—405. Available from: http://dx.doi.org/10.1148/radiology.183.2.1561340.

[2] Ferreira S, Jhingran SG, Johnson PC. Radionuclide cisternography for the study of arachnoid cysts: a case report. Neuroradiology 1980;19(3):167—9.

[3] Tali ET, Ercan N, Kaymaz M, Pasaoglu A, Jinkins JR. Intrathecal gadolinium (gado-pentetate dimeglumine)-enhanced MR cisternography used to determine potential communication between the cerebrospinal fluid pathways and intracranial arachnoid cysts. Neuroradiology 2004;46(9):744—54. Available from: http://dx.doi.org/10.1007/s00234-004-1240-0.

[4] Wolpert SM, Scott RM. The value of metrizamide CT cisternography in the management of cerebral arachnoid cysts. AJNR Am J Neuroradiol 1981;2(1):29—35.

[5] Kanda T, Nakai Y, Oba H, Toyoda K, Kitajima K, Furui S. Gadolinium deposition in the brain. Magn Reson Imaging 2016;34(10):1346—50. Available from: http://dx.doi.org/10.1016/j.mri.2016.08.024.

[6] Al-Holou WN, Terman S, Kilburg C, Garton HJ, Muraszko KM, Maher CO. Prevalence and natural history of arachnoid cysts in adults. J Neurosurg 2013;118 (2):222—31. Available from: http://dx.doi.org/10.3171/2012.10.JNS12548.

[7] de Oliveira RS, Amato MC, Santos MV, Simao GN, Machado HR. Extradural arachnoid cysts in children. Childs Nerv Syst 2007;23(11):1233—8. Available from: http://dx.doi.org/10.1007/s00381-007-0414-6.

[8] Petridis AK, Doukas A, Barth H, Mehdorn HM. Spinal cord compression caused by idiopathic intradural arachnoid cysts of the spine: review of the literature and illustrated case. Eur Spine J 2010;19(Suppl 2):S124—9. Available from: http://dx.doi.org/10.1007/s00586-009-1156-9.

[9] Maiuri F, Iaconetta G, Gangemi M. Arachnoid cyst of the lateral ventricle. Surg Neurol 1997;48(4):401—4.

[10] Awaji M, Okamoto K, Nishiyama K. Magnetic resonance cisternography for preoperative evaluation of arachnoid cysts. Neuroradiology 2007;49(9):721—6. Available from: http://dx.doi.org/10.1007/s00234-007-0248-7.

[11] De Keersmaecker B, Ramaekers P, Claus F, Witters I, Ortibus E, Naulaers G, et al. Outcome of 12 antenatally diagnosed fetal arachnoid cysts: case series and review of the literature. Eur J Paediatr Neurol 2015;19(2):114−21. Available from: http://dx.doi.org/10.1016/j.ejpn.2014.12.008.

[12] Osborn AG, Preece MT. Intracranial cysts: radiologic-pathologic correlation and imaging approach. Radiology 2006;239(3):650−64. Available from: http://dx.doi.org/10.1148/radiol.2393050823.

[13] Tsuruda JS, Chew WM, Moseley ME, Norman D. Diffusion-weighted MR imaging of the brain: value of differentiating between extraaxial cysts and epidermoid tumors. AJNR Am J Neuroradiol 1990;11(5):925−31 discussion 932−924.

[14] Tubbs RS, Salter EG, Oakes WJ. Neurenteric cyst: case report and a review of the potential dysembryology. Clin Anat 2006;19(7):669−72. Available from: http://dx.doi.org/10.1002/ca.20204.

[15] Yildiz H, Erdogan C, Yalcin R, Yazici Z, Hakyemez B, Parlak M, et al. Evaluation of communication between intracranial arachnoid cysts and cisterns with phase-contrast cine MR imaging. AJNR Am J Neuroradiol 2005;26(1):145−51.

[16] Chalela JA, Kidwell CS, Nentwich LM, Luby M, Butman JA, Demchuk AM, et al. Magnetic resonance imaging and computed tomography in emergency assessment of patients with suspected acute stroke: a prospective comparison. Lancet 2007;369 (9558):293−8 http://dx.doi.org/10.1016/S0140-6736(07)60151-2.

[17] Mittal S, Wu Z, Neelavalli J, Haacke EM. Susceptibility-weighted imaging: technical aspects and clinical applications, part 2. AJNR Am J Neuroradiol 2009;30(2):232−52. Available from: http://dx.doi.org/10.3174/ajnr.A1461.

[18] Helland CA, Wester K. A population based study of intracranial arachnoid cysts: clinical and neuroimaging outcomes following surgical cyst decompression in adults. J Neurol Neurosurg Psychiatry 2007;78(10):1129−35. Available from: http://dx.doi.org/10.1136/jnnp.2006.107995.

[19] Helland CA, Wester K. A population-based study of intracranial arachnoid cysts: clinical and neuroimaging outcomes following surgical cyst decompression in children. J Neurosurg 2006;105(Suppl 5):385−90. Available from: http://dx.doi.org/10.3171/ped.2006.105.5.385.

15

Arachnoid Cyst—Prenatal Detection, Management, and Perinatal Outcome

Bart De Keersmaecker[1,2], Michael Aertsen[1], Liesbeth Thewissen[1], Katrien Jansen[1] and Luc De Catte[1]

[1]UZ Leuven Hospitals, Leuven, Belgium [2]AZ Groeninge Hospital, Kortrijk, Belgium

Arachnoid Cysts: Epidemiology, Biology, and Neuroimaging
DOI: http://dx.doi.org/10.1016/B978-0-12-809932-2.00015-6

ABBREVIATIONS

AC	arachnoid cyst
ADHD	attention deficit hyperactivity disorder
CC	corpus callosum
CNS	central nervous system
CSF	cerebrospinal fluid
CPS	cystoperitoneal shunting
MRI	magnetic resonance imaging
VPS	ventriculoperitoneal shunting

RECOMMENDATIONS—LEVEL OF EVIDENCE

Level I

There is no Level I evidence available concerning prenatal detection of arachnoid cysts (ACs) by ultrasound or magnetic resonance imaging (MRI) that improves the perinatal outcome.

Level II

Fetal ACs are occasionally associated with chromosomal abnormalities. The presence of associated structural defects should prompt cytogenetic evaluation.

Fetal MRI improves the visualization of associated central nervous system anomalies.

BACKGROUND

ACs in the newborn are rare, usually benign lesions, representing 1% of all intracranial masses and about 1% of the space occupying lesions in childhood [1,2]. They result from an abnormal development of the leptomeningae. The arachnoid space is created by the expansion of the extracellular space of the loose primitive mesenchyme, which early in fetal life surrounds the neural tube. The outer layer of cells forms the arachnoid web and the inner layer, the pia mater. The intervening space is filled by fine trabeculae [1]. Abnormal splitting of these layers and entrapment of cerebrospinal fluid (CSF) causes ACs to develop [3,4]. Their content is similar but not equal to CSF [3]. They can originate from trauma, meningitis, and hemorrhage and usually communicate with the arachnoid space [1].

AC are located throughout brain near the surface and in proximity to the arachnoid cisterns at the level of the main fissures and the sella tursica [4–8]. Most of the ACs are located supratentorially; 50% are located in the middle cranial fossa. They are also found in the quadrigeminal cistern (5%–10%), suprasellar cistern (5%–10%), cerebral convexity (5%), or posterior fossa (5%–10%) [2,4,8]. The volume effect of the cyst on the adjacent brain may interfere with normal neural processes crucial for the development of the brain and thereby give rise to permanent, irreversible learning difficulties and behavioral problems [9]. AC often occur as isolated lesions but an association with dysgenesis of the corpus callosum and ventriculomegaly has been described [10]. In these cases, interhemispheric ACs represent more a developmental anomaly in the spectrum of corpus callosum agenesis [11] rather than a true AC.

ULTRASOUND DIAGNOSIS

Congenital ACs are diagnosed frequently on routine mid-trimester ultrasound as hypoechoic masses without color Doppler signal. They are well-delineated, unilocular, and regularly shaped and usually single in origin located on the surface of the brain, and may create a mass effect. Supratentorial ACs are picked up later in gestation than the ones in posterior fossa [12]. Diagnosis of ACs in a recent large series was made in 25% of the cases in the second trimester while the remaining 75% were diagnosed between 28 and 34 weeks of gestation [12]. First trimester diagnosis of an AC in the posterior fossa has been made by transvaginal ultrasound as early as 13 weeks of gestation [13]. Most ACs remain stable in size during pregnancy. Elbers reported even a spontaneously resolving AC at 32 weeks of gestation [7].

Fetal ACs are occasionally associated with chromosomal abnormalities but only the presence of an associated structural defect should prompt cytogenetic evaluation. The incidence of associated chromosomal abnormalities is estimated at 6% but fetuses with isolated cysts are euploid [14]. Various associated chromosomal abnormalities have been reported: trisomies 8,13,18,20 [15,16]. AC may also be associated with single gene mutuations (Xq22, 9q22, 14q32.3,11p15), or be part of syndromal malformations, such as Aicardi syndrome, Chudley Mc Cullough syndrome, neurofibromatosis type I, Marfan's syndrome, and autosomal dominant polycystic kidney disease [15,17–26]. In bilateral AC, glutaric aciduria type 1 has to be excluded [27] (Fig. 15.1).

AC should be differentiated from porencephalic cysts which are usually unilateral, communicate with the lateral ventricular system, and lack the mass effect because they result from infarction or another destructive brain lesion [28]. Interhemispheric cysts are usually centered

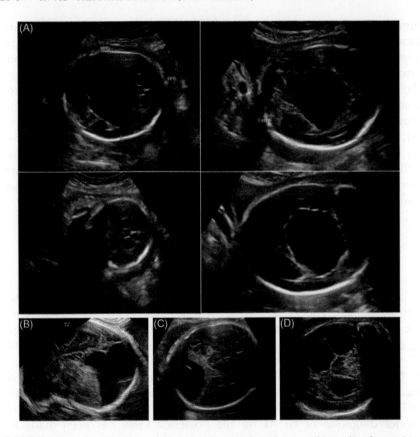

FIGURE 15.1   (A) Series of axial views of an arachnoid cyst at 28 weeks of gestation. The AC measures $32 \times 37 \times 37$ mm and compresses the midcerebral structures, pons, and cerebellum. The corpus callosum is compressed and bilateral ventriculomegaly is present. (B) Suprasellar arachnoid cyst at 32 weeks of gestation without associated anomalies. (C) Arachnoid cyst of the posterior fossa at 30 weeks of gestation. (D) Axial view of a fetal head at 32 weeks of gestation demonstrating multiple ACs without sonographic evidence of compression of the parenchyma.

at the midline. The asymmetric ventriculomegaly is often the most obvious feature. Choroid plexus cysts, commonly found in the lateral ventricles on a second trimester scan [29], usually resolve by 26 weeks of gestation. Glioependymal cysts are located in the parenchyma of the brain and have an ependymal lining with ciliated cells staining with antibodies against glial fibrillary acidic protein [30]. Occasionally they occur in association with agenesis of the corpus callosum [31,32]. Aneurysms of the vein of Galen and other vascular anomalies are easily differentiated from other brain lesions by color Doppler analysis. Other rare conditions to differentiate are schizencephaly, craniopharyngioma, benign cystic gliomas, Rathke cleft cysts, cystic astrocytoma, colloid cyst of the third ventricle, teratoma, and intraventricular hemorrhage. Differential diagnosis of ACs in the posterior fossa includes megacisterna magna, Blake Pouch cysts, and Dandy Walker malformation [33,34].

Fetal MRI improves the visualization of associated central nervous system abnormalities such as heterotopia, corpus callosum dysgenesis, compression of the aqueduct, and the differentiation with other cystic

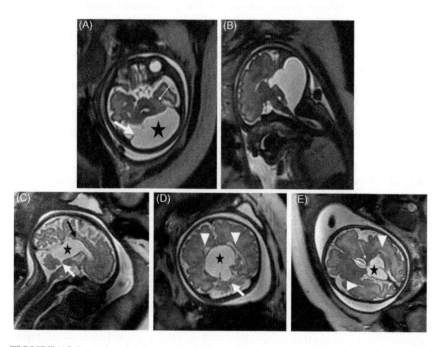

FIGURE 15.2   (A) Axial T2-weighted image demonstrating a large retrocerebellar cyst (star) with clear depiction of the cyst wall (thick white arrow). The cyst is causing displacement of the left superficial cerebellar hemisphere anteriorly (thin white arrow). (B) Sagittal T2-weighted image of a the same large retrocerebellar cyst (star) causing mass effect on the vermis (black arrowhead). The vermis appears complete with full coverage of the fourth ventricle. Additional secondary cranial displacement of the tentorium (thick white arrow). (C) Mid-sagittal T2-weighted image demonstrating a large midline interhemispheric cyst (star) cranial of the cerebellum and posterior of the quadrigeminal plate and basal ganglia. Caudally there is mass effect of the cyst on the cranial aspect of the cerebellum (thick white arrow) and cranially there is superior displacement of the splenium of the corpus callosum (thick black arrow). (D) Coronal T2-weighted image of the large midline interhemispheric cyst (star) cranial of the cerebellum causing mild mass effect on the vermis and superficial parts of the cerebellar hemispheres, No secondary dilatation of the lateral ventricles (white arrowheads). (E) Axial T2-weighted image at the level of the basal ganglia and third ventricle. The cranial part of the cyst is causing some mass effect on the posterior aspect of the basal ganglia of the deep hemisphere. Discrete bulging of the wall of the third ventricle indicating discrete dilatation (curved lines). No dilatation of the lateral ventricles (white arrowheads).

lesions. Of the 48 reported ACs, 24 underwent a prenatal MRI which confirmed the prenatal ultrasound of AC without additional findings in only seven cases [10,13,18,19,33,35−52]. In the other seven cases of AC, dysgenesis was found on MRI. In one patient, multiple ACs compressed the temporal lobe and the splenium of the corpus callosum, which was not appreciated either by prenatal ultrasound nor prenatal MRI but was only picked up by postnatal MRI [10]. In a meta-analysis, two cases of callosal abnormalities were missed at the ultrasound scan, but picked up at fetal MRI while two other anomalies were only detected at postnatal examination consisting of agenesis of the corpus callosum in one case and a teratoma and agenesis of the corpus callosum in the other case [14] (Fig. 15.2).

The prognosis of a fetus with an AC depends particularly on the brain integrity rather than on the volume or location of the cyst [22]. The presence of a normal corpus callosum, absence of extra-CNS anomalies and ventriculomegaly, a slowly growing cyst, and a location near the Sylvian fissure are favorable variables.

Perinatal management of fetuses with AC compares with fetuses without structural defects. However, association with macrocephaly may lead to cephalopelvic disproportion for which a C-section is indicated.

POSTNATAL WORKUP

Prenatally diagnosed AC should be explored carefully by clinical evaluation of the neonate in order to exclude associated cerebral and extracerebral congenital anomalies and to distinguish between isolated AC or not. Special attention should be paid to head circumference, signs and symptoms of raised intracranial pressure with examination of the fundi, abnormal bulging of the skull, and visual and neuroendocrine symptoms. In particular suprasellar, quadrigeminal, and interhemispheric AC may cause hydrocephalus due to unilateral or bilateral obstruction of CSF flow prenatally, in the first weeks or later in life. Compression of the optic nerve, the pituitary gland or stalk and hypothalamic structures have been described as well [3]. Neonatal imaging consists of trans fontanel brain ultrasound and MRI examination, if not performed prenatally, to exclude associated cerebral abnormalities and to confirm the lesion (location, side, size of the cyst). Heterotopia, cortical malformations, polymicrogyria, abnormalities in the white matter and a- or dysgenesis of the corpus callosum will be important determinants for outcome. If not performed prenatally, associated brain abnormalities should prompt cytogenetic evaluation.

OUTCOME OF ARACHNOID CYSTS

The natural history of AC varies extensively: regression, stabilization, slow growth towards acute enlargement of cyst, subdural effusion following rupture of cyst, and subdural or intracystic bleeding, with or without history of trauma. Outcome of isolated ACs is generally good. Most cysts remain clinically silent and are detected incidentally.

The widespread use of computed tomography, MRI, and ultrasound scans for neurological symptoms, such as headache, developmental delay, epilepsy, or neuropsychological dysfunction, leads to an increased detection rate of clinically nonrelated AC and shift in age distribution towards the early years of life in the absence of cyst-related symptoms [53]. If the cyst itself produces symptoms, the neurological signs reflect the anatomical localization and the effect on CSF flow; however, an AC with associated abnormalities may give rise to symptoms irrespective of the cyst itself. The neurodevelopmental prognosis depends particularly on the brain integrity rather than the cyst itself.

The AC growth and localization determine largely the need for postnatal surgery. The supratentorial cysts, suprasellar cysts, posterior fossa cysts, and quadrigeminal cistern cysts can give rise to hydrocephalus and macrocephaly. Visual impairment or loss and hypothalamic–pituitary dysfunction has been documented in suprasellar cysts, whereas motor development disorders are associated with cysts in the region of the third ventricle. In addition, hemorrhagic complications of ACs are common, and occur ipsilateral to ACs of the middle fossa. Interhemispheric cysts in particular may be associated with corpus callosal dysgenesis, and as such are considered part of a developmental aberration. Although some of these cysts are arachnoid in origin, others are probably neuroectodermal cysts. In temporal lobe ACs an underlying maldevelopment of the cortex may be present, resulting more frequently in attention deficit hyperactivity disorder and speech problems. In other patients with seizures the relationship with intracranial ACs remains unclear [54,55].

SURGERY

The large majority of ACs do not require surgery. In a systematic review, hydrocephaly and mass effect on the adjacent structures were observed in 23% [14] necessitating surgery in 34.7%. While surgery in children with raised intracranial pressure or local symptomatology related to the cyst is clearly indicated, preventive surgery or surgical intervention for other clinical symptoms such as headache, developmental delay, epilepsy, or neuropsychological dysfunction remains controversial [3,15,56].

Literature is often biased by describing only the subgroup of patients sent in for surgery. In a recent prospective long-term survey of 27 children from the age of 2 months up to 17 years, a restrictive attitude to surgery for intracranial ACs in the absence of objectively verified symptoms and signs or obstructions of CSF pathways was advocated. No clinical improvement was found in relation with an objective radiological assessment of reduction of the cyst volume [56]. A follow-up study of 19 children with a conservative management of supratentorial AC, failed to show a correlation between size of the cyst and severity of neurological symptoms.

The diagnosis of AC as an incidental finding at birth without neurological impairment, or with a neurological deficit unrelated to the cyst's location, warrants a careful follow-up in the first 2 years of life. Children with a prenatal diagnosis of isolated AC were more likely to experience symptoms or having surgery in the first 25 months of life, while occurrence of symptoms was relatively unlikely thereafter [14]. A patient with neurological deficit and space occupying lesions explaining the symptomatology or the raised intracranial pressure, is eligible for surgery.

Debate in the literature exists between ventriculoperitoneal shunting (VPS) or cystoperitoneal shunting (CPS) in cases of hydrocephalus, and open microsurgical/endoscopic fenestration with cystoventriculostomy or cystocisternostomy [15]. However, CPS is associated with several complications, including CSF overdrainage or shunt dependency rendering the efficacy of CPS as an initial treatment for AC questionable [57], see Chapter 12, Shunt Techniques—Cystoperitoneal Shunt and Chapter 14, Overdrainage Syndromes in Shunted Arachnoid Cysts, both of Volume 2.

Progress in neuroendoscopic instruments and techniques made cysts fenestration the primary therapeutic procedure. However, due to a high rate of complications, strict indications are recommended for fenestration surgery in AC [58].

If hydrocephalus is marked or progressive after fenestration, a shunt may be inserted.

SUMMARY

Slow growth of the AC, absence of ventriculomegaly, location near the Sylvian fissure, the presence of a normal corpus callosum, and the absence of additional central nervous system anomalies are favorable variables that can be used in prenatal counseling.

Large prospective studies with standardized protocols for diagnosis and management are needed in order to further ascertain the rate of abnormal neurodevelopmental outcome in children with a prenatal diagnosis of isolated intracranial cysts.

If surgery is indicated, cysts fenestration is considered the primary procedure.

References

[1] Timor-Trisch I, Monteguado A, Cohen A. Ultrasonography of the prenatal and neonatal brain. In : Appleton and Lange, Fetal Neurosonography of Congenital Brain Anomalies, Stamford, Connecticut 1996:147−219.

[2] Di Rocco C, Caldarelli M. Supratentorial interhemispheric and pineal region cysts. In: Ralmondi AJ, Choux M, Di Rocco C, editors. Intracranial cyst lesions, 153−68. New York: Springer Verlag; 1993. p. 529−30.

[3] Westmaier T, Schweitzer T, Ernestus RI. Arachnoid cysts. Adv Exp Med Biol 2012;724:37−50.

[4] Hayward R. Postnatal management and outcome for fetal-diagnosed intra-cerebral cystic masses and tumours. Prenat Diagn 2009;29(4):396−401. Available from: http://dx.doi.org/10.1002/pd.2152.

[5] Basaldella L, Orvieto E, Dei Tos AP, Della Barbera M, Valente M, Longatti P. Causes of arachnoid cyst development and expansion. Neurosurg Focus 2007;22(2):E4.

[6] Cincu R, Agrawal A, Eiras J. Intracranial arachnoid cysts: current concepts and treatment alternatives. Clin Neurol Neurosurg 2007;109(10):837−43. Available from: http://dx.doi.org/10.1016/j.clineuro.2007.07.013.

[7] Pascual-Castroviejo I, Roche M, Martinez Bermejo A, Arcas J, Garcia Blasquez M. Primary intracranial arachnoid cysts. A study of 67 childhood cases. Childs Nerv system 1991;7:257−63.

[8] Wester K. Peculiarities of intracranial arachnoid cysts : location, sidedness and sex distribution in 126 consecutive patients. Neurosurgery 1999;45:775−9.

[9] Wester K. Intracranial arachnoid cyst-do they impair mental function. J Neurol 2008;255(8):1113−20.

[10] Blaicher W, Prayer D, Kuhle S, Deutinger J, Bernachek G. Combined prenatal ultrasound and magnetic resonance imaging in two fetuses with suspected arachnoid cyst. Ultrasound Obstet Gynecol 2001;18(2):166−8.

[11] Barkovich AJ, Simon EM, Walsh CA. Callosal agenesis with cyst: a better understanding and new classification. Neurology 2001;56(2):220−7.

[12] De Keersmaecker B, Ramaekers P, Claus F, Witters I, Ortibus E, Naulaers G, et al. Outcome of 12 antenatally diagnosed fetal arachnoid cysts: case series and review of the literature. Eur J Paediatr Neurol 2015 Mar;19(2):114−21 http://dx.doi.org/10.1016/j.ejpn.2014.12.008. Epub 2014 Dec 27.

[13] Bretelle F, Senat M, Bernard J, Hillion Y, Ville Y. First trimester diagnosis of fetal arachnoid cyst: prenatal implication. Ultrasound Obstet Gynecol 2002;20:400−2.

[14] Youssef A, D'Antonio F, Khalil A, Papageorghiou A, Ciardulli A, Lanzone E, et al. Outcome of fetuses with supratentorial extra-axial intracranial cysts. A systematic review. Fetal Diagn ther 2016;40:1−12.

[15] Ali ZS, Lang SS, Bakar D, Storm PB, Stein SC. Pediatric intracranial arachnoid cysts: comparative effectiveness of surgical treatment options. Childs Nerv Syst 2014;30(3) 461−46.

[16] Chapman T, Perez FA, Ishak GE, Doherty D. Prenatal diagnosis of Chudley-McCullough syndrome. Am J Med Genet A 2016 Sep;170(9):2426−30 http://dx.doi.org/10.1002/ajmg.a.37806. Epub 2016 Jun 17.

[17] Alehan FK, Gurakan B, Agildere M. Familial arachnoid cysts in association with autosomal dominant polycystic kidney disease. Pediatrics 2002;110(1 Pt 1):e13.

[18] Pilu G, Falco A, Sandri F, Cocchi G, Ancora G, Bovicelli L. Differential diagnosis and outcome of fetal intracranial hypoechoic lesions: report of 21 cases. Ultrasound Obstet Gynecol 1997;9:229−36.

[19] Souter V, Glass I, Chapman D, Raff M, Parisi M, Opheim K, et al. Multiple fetal anomalies associated with subte subtelomeric chromosomal rearrangements. Ultrasound Obstet Gynecol 2003;21:609−15.

[20] Chen C, Suh Y, Weng S, Tsai F, Chen C, Liu Y, et al. Rapid aneuploidy diagnosis of trisomy 18 by array comparative genomic hybridization using uncultured amniocytes in a pregnancy with fetal arachnoid cyst detected in late second trimester. Taiwanese J Obstetrics Gynecol 2012;51 481e48.

[21] Stein QP, Boyle JG, Crotwell PL, Flanagan JD, Johnson KJ, Davis- Keppen L. Prenatally diagnosed trisomy 20 mosaicism associated with arachnoid cyst of basal cistern. Prenat Diagn 2008;28:e1169−70.

[22] Al-Holou W, Yew A, Boomsaad Z, Garton H, Muraszko K, Maher C. Prevalence and natural history of arachnoid cysts in children. J Neurosurg Pediatrics 2010;5 057008−050850.

[23] Bannister C, Russell S, Rimmer S, Mowie D. Fetal arachnoid cysts: their site, progress, prognosis and differential diagnosis. Eur J Pediatr Surg 1999;9:27−8.

[24] Napolitano R, Maruotti G, Quarantelli M, Martinelli P, Paladini D. Prenatal diagnosis of Seckel Syndrome on 3-D Dimensional Sonography and Magnetic Resonance imaging. J Ultrasound Med 2009;28:369−74.

[25] Dror R, Malinger G, Ben-Sira L, Lev D, Pick C, Lerman Sagie T. Developmental outcome of children with enlargement of the cistern magna identified in utero. J Child Neurol 2009;24(12):1486−92.

[26] Martinez-Lage J, Poza M, Rodriguez C. Bilateral temporal arachnoid cyst in neurofibromatosis. J Child Neurol 1993;8:383−5.

[27] Lutcherath V, Waaler PE, Jellum E, Wester K. Children with bilateral temporal arachnoid cysts may have glutaric aciduria type 1 (GAT1); operation without knowing that may be harmful. Acta Neurochir (Wien) 2000;142(9):1025−30.

[28] Abergel A, Lacolm A, Massoud M, Massardier J, des Portes V, Guibaud L. Expanding porencephalic cysts: prenatal imaging and differential diagnosis. Fetal Diagn Ther 2016 Jul 14; (ehead of print).

[29] Gross S, Shulman L, Tolley E. Isolated fetal choroid plexus cysts and trisomy 18: a review and meta-analysis. AJOG 1995;172:83−7.

[30] Inoue T, Matsushima T, Fukui M, Iwaki T, Takeshita I, Kuromatsu C. Immunohistochemical study of intracranial cysts. Neurosurgery 1988;23(5):576−81.

[31] Tange Y, Aoki K, Mori K, Niijima S, Maeda M. Interhemispheric glioependymal cyst with agenesis of corpus callosum- case report. Neur Med Chir 2000;40(10):536−42.

[32] Muhler M, Hartmann C, Werner W, Meyer O, Bollman R, Klingebiel R. Fetal MRI demonstrates glioependymal cyst in a case of sonographic unilateral ventriculomegaly. Pediatr Radiol 2007;37(4):391−5.

[33] Gandolfi Colleoni G, Contro E, Carletti A, Ghi T, Campobasso G, Rembouskos G, et al. Prenatal diagnosis and outcome of fetal posterior fossa fluid collections. Ultrasound Obstet Gynecol 2012;39(6):625−31 http://dx.doi.org/10.1002/uog. 11071. Epub 2012 May 14.

[34] Nelson D, Maher K, Gilles F. A different approach to cysts of the posterior fossa. Pediatric Neurology 2004;34:720−32.

[35] Elbers S, Furness M. Resolution of presumed arachnoid cyst in utero. Ultrasound Obstet Gynecol 1999;14:353−5.

[36] Hogge W, Schnatterly P, Ferguson 2nd J. Early prenatal diagnosis of an infratentorial arachnoid cyst : association with an unbalanced translocation. Prenat Diagn 1995;15:186−8.

[37] Diakoumakis E, Weinberg B, Mollin J. Prenatal sonographic diagnosis of suprasellar arachnoid cyst. J Ultrasound Med 1986;5:529−30.

[38] Meizner I, Barki Y, Tadmor R, Katz M. In utero ultrasonic detection of fetal arachnoid cyst. J Clin Ultrasound 1988;16:509.

[39] Raman S, Rachagan S, Lim C. Prenatal diagnosis of a fossa posterior cyst. J Clin Ultrasound 1991;19:434−7.

[40] Langer B, Haddad J, Favre R, Frigue V, Schlaeder G. Fetal arachnoid cyst: report of two cases. Ultrasound Obstet Gynecol 1994;4:68−72.

[41] Hassan J, Sepulveda W, Teixeira J, Cox P. Glioependymal and arachnoid cysts : unusual cases of early ventriculomegaly in utero. Prenat Diagn 1996;16:729−33.

[42] Rafferty P, Britton J, Penna L, Ville Y. Prenatal diagnosis of a large fetal arachnoid cyst. Ultrasound Obstet Gynecol 1998;12:358−61.

[43] Levine D, Barnes P, Madsen J, Abbott J, Mehta T, Edelmann R. Central nervous system abnormalities assessed with prenatal magnetic resonance imaging. Obstet Gyn 1999;94:1011−19.

[44] Golash A, Mitchell G, Mallucci C, Pilling D. Prenatal diagnosis of suprasellar arachnoid cyst and postnatal endoscopic treatment. Childs Nerv System 2001;17:739−42.

[45] Nakamura Y, Mizukuwa K, Yamamoto K, Nagashima T. Endoscopic treatment for a huge neonatal prepontine-suprasellar arachnoid cyst: a case report. Pediatric Neurosurg 2001;35.

[46] Kusuka Y, Luedemann W, Oi S, Schwardfegar R, Samii M. Fetal arachnoid cyst of the quadrigemal cistern in MRI and ultrasound. Child Nerv Syst 2005;21:1065−6.

[47] Fujimura J, Shima Y, Arai H, Ogawa R, Fukunaga Y. Management of a suprasellar arachnoid cyst identified using prenatal sonography. J Clin Ultrasound 2006;34:92−4.

[48] Chen C. Prenatal diagnosis of Arachnoid cysts. Taiwan J Obstet 2007;46(1):87−197.

[49] Haino K, Serikawa T, Kikuchi A, Takakuwa K, Tanaka K. Prenatal diagnosis of fetal arachnoid cyst of the quadrigeminal cistern in ultrasonography and MRI. Prenat Diagn 2009;29(11):1078−80. Available from: http://dx.doi.org/10.1002/pd.2346.

[50] Coutinho L, Fan Y, Inocencio G, Sousa R, Dias C, Ferreira L. Arachnoid cyst of posterior fossa : a case report. Ultrasound Obstet Gynecol 2010;36(suppl. 1):186.

[51] Gedikbasi A, Palabiyik F, Oztarhan A, Yildirim G, Eren C, Ozyurt S, et al. Prenatal diagnosis of a suprasellar arachnoid cyst with 2-and 3 dimensional sonography and fetal magnetic resonance imaging: difficulties in management and review of the literature. J Ultrasound Med 2010;29(10):1487−93.

[52] Tang P, Chang K, Hwang W, Yeo S, Ong S. Fetal hypothalamic hamartoma with suprasellar arachnoid cyst. Ultrasound Obstet Gynecol 2012;40(6):725−6 http://dx.doi.org/10.1002/uog.11145. Epub 2012 nov 26.

[53] Gosalakkal JA. Intracranial arachnoid cysts in children: a review of pathogenesis, clinical features, and management. Pediatr Neurol 2002;26(2):93−8.

[54] Griebel ML, Williams JP, Russell SS, Spence GT, Glasier CM. Clinical and developmental findings in children with giant interhemispheric cysts and dysgenesis of the corpus callosum. Pediatr Neurol. 1995 Sep;13(2):119−24.

[55] Haverkamp F, Heep A, Woelfle J. Psychomotor development in children with early diagnosed giant interhemispheric cysts. Dev Med Child Neurol 2002 Aug;44(8):556−60.

[56] Rabiei K, Högfeldt MJ, Doria-Medina R, Tisell M. Surgery for intracranial arachnoid cysts in children—a prospective long-term study. Child's Nervous System 2016;1−7 http://dx.doi.org/10.1007/s00381-016-3064-89. doi:10.1007/s00381-013-2306-2.

[57] Martinez-Lage JF, Ruiz-Espejo AM, Almagro MJ, Alfaro R, Felipe-Murcia M, Lopez-Guerrero AL. CSF overdrainage in shunted intracranial arachnoid cysts: a series and review. Childs Nerv Syst 2009;25(9):1061−9. Available from: http://dx.doi.org/10.1007/s00381-009-0910-y.

[58] Choi JW, Lee JY, Phi JH, Kim SK, Wang KC. Stricter indications are recommended for fenestration surgery in intracranial arachnoid cysts of children. Childs Nerv Syst 2015;31(1):77−86. Available from: http://dx.doi.org/10.1007/s00381-014-2525-1.

SPECT Studies in Patients With Arachnoid Cysts

Juan F. Martínez-Lage[1,2], María-José Almagro[1] and Antonio L. López-Guerrero[1,2]

[1]Virgen de la Arrixaca University Hospital, Murcia, Spain [2]University of Murcia Medical School, Murcia, Spain

O U T L I N E

Arachnoid Cysts: Epidemiology, Biology, and Neuroimaging
DOI: http://dx.doi.org/10.1016/B978-0-12-809932-2.00016-8

199

ABBREVIATIONS

AC	arachnoid cyst
CBF	cerebral blood flow
CSF	cerebrospinal fluid
CT	computerized tomography
ICP	intracranial pressure
MRI	magnetic resonance imaging
PET	positron emission tomography
rCBF	regional blood flow
SPECT	single-photon emission computerized tomography

INTRODUCTION

Most publications concerning the use of single-photon emission computerized tomography (SPECT) correspond to levels of evidence IV (case study, case series) or V (single expert opinion or review of expert opinion). An arachnoid cyst (AC) is a pouch that contains a fluid similar to cerebrospinal fluid (CSF) and that is usually of congenital origin [1]. Most ACs manifest before the age of 10 years, especially during the first 3 years of life [1]. Exceptionally they become symptomatic during adolescence and adulthood [1]. Formerly, ACs were exclusively discovered after diagnostic workup motivated by the patients' clinical manifestations. Nowadays, the cysts are also revealed by a neuroimaging study carried out for reasons unrelated to the cyst, as happens in the assessment of a head injury, epilepsy, or headaches [1]. The lesions are then denominated *incidental arachnoid cysts*. At the time of obtaining the clinical history, it is evident that some symptoms were previously present but the patients seem to have ignored or underestimated them.

Most diagnostic methods, such as ultrasound (US), computerized tomography (CT), and magnetic resonance imaging (MRI), depict only *anatomical* details, such as site, size, and relationships of the ACs. CT-cisternography reveals the existence of a communication of the cysts with the cisterns and/or subarachnoid spaces; information that may help in choosing the treatment modality. The classification of middle fossa ACs [2] into three types is based on data regarding size, shape, and degree of communication of the cysts. Sato et al. [3] also utilized CT-cisternography to describe a morphological classification of middle fossa ACs of practical interest. The cysts are classified as anteromedial and anterolateral. Anteromedial cysts have a tongue of cerebral tissue that acts as an obstacle for establishing a surgical communication of the cysts with the basilar cisterns. In anterolateral lesions the tongue of brain parenchyma is situated superficially and does not obstruct the surgical route towards the suprasellar and prepontine cisterns.

Obviously, ACs that exert pressure on the surrounding brain tissue or obstruct the CSF pathways producing hydrocephalus need no further diagnostic tests for indicating surgical treatment [1]. The role of hydrocephalus in patients with ACs and its indications for surgery has been amply discussed elsewhere (e.g., see Ref. [4]). However there exist cases of doubtful indications of surgery that require performing further diagnostic tests to detect an eventual brain dysfunction [5–7].

Functional studies, including electroencephalography (EEG), neurophysiological testing, neuropsychological exams [7], functional MRI, and intracranial pressure (ICP) recording [8], have all been utilized in the evaluation of intracranial ACs. As some ACs evolve with epilepsy, *magneto-encephalography* has been used to localize the seizure focus in a 36-year-old woman patient with an abnormal pachygyric cortex not seen by MRI, that was initially attributed to a large AC of the parietal convexity [9]. Positron emission tomography (PET) has also been utilized in the evaluation of ACs [10–12]. PET is a tool devised for the detection of pathological conditions that cause metabolic impairment of the brain.

SPECT is often used for assessing cerebral perfusion changes in several conditions, such as head trauma, epilepsy, dementia, and cerebrovascular diseases. SPECT is a method of nuclear medicine that uses pharmaceuticals with specific bound isotopes and is commonly used for assessing regional cerebral blood flow (rCBF). In addition, SPECT can also detect subtle deterioration in brain function. However, cerebral SPECT has been scarcely utilized for the study of ACs, as attested by the few reports that have addressed its use in these lesions [3,13–15]. In addition, most publications consist of single case reports [16–21].

Although not yet put into practice, SPECT studies could also be utilized in cases of cyst overshunting, to detect subtle deterioration when shunt removal is planned. The information provided by both anatomical and functional diagnostic tests can also help in choosing the most appropriate type of treatment (observation or surgical) and in deciding the most convenient surgical strategy (shunting, craniotomy, or neuroendoscopy procedures) [22]. In the present chapter, an update of cerebral SPECT in the study of ACs will be briefly discussed, including a review of the relevant publications on the subject.

PATIENTS AND METHODS

An Elscint SP4 camera was used for performing cerebral SPECT scanning in our study. The equipment incorporates a padded headrest to aid in patient's head immobilization. The individuals are given

25 mCi of mTc-HMPAO intravenously and then they are introduced into the camera and placed supine. Pediatric patients are either reassured or premedicated with oral pentobarbital or midazolam if necessary, given the importance of maintaining a still position of the head during the study. The dosage of radiotracer in children is adjusted to their body weight 0.2–0.3 mCi/kg (maximum of 3–5 mCi). For each SPECT scanning, 60 images of 30 seconds each are obtained, which gives a total count of approximately 5 million points. Each image is acquired every 6 degrees over 360 degrees. To increase image resolution and point counting, the smallest radius of rotation is chosen. Image reconstructions are performed following the sagittal, axial, and coronal planes. To improve the visibility of the results, the images are automatically colored using a numerically based scale that denotes the degree of the radiotracer uptake. Each SPECT scanning study takes approximately 30 minutes.

A previous study from our institution gathered demographic, clinical, and neuroimaging data of 20 consecutive patients previously diagnosed with intracranial ACs [15]. Data pertaining to the mode of presentation (symptomatic or asymptomatic), modality of treatment (observation or surgery), and outcomes were analyzed as well. The group consisted of patients with ACs located at the sylvian fissure ($n = 11$), the posterior fossa ($n = 4$), the cerebral midline ($n = 2$), and the ventricles ($n = 3$). The cyst size was estimated by the formula $(a + b + c)/3$, with a, b, and c being the value of the diameter of the lesion in the three axes of the space. The formula represented the mean diameter of the cyst. The lesions were divided according to the length of the mean axis in two groups: <3 cm and >3 cm, aimed at correlating the results with the cysts' size. Our study focused mainly on the 11 patients with ACs located at the sylvian fissure for two reasons. Firstly, we presupposed that Acs in this location should readily manifest local signs of cerebral hypoperfusion given their proximity to major cerebral arteries. Secondly, the subgroup of sylvian Acs was the most numerous, which would strengthen the validity of the survey.

The study results were classified in two broad categories regarding isotope uptake: normal or decreased. *Empty images* of radiotracer were not taken into consideration for the purpose of the investigation as they corresponded to the vacuum image of isotope uptake left by the bulk of the cyst. When there was a decrease in the count of a determined cerebral region showing an asymmetry greater than 10% as compared with its contralateral brain zone, it was regarded as decreased rCBF. In posterior fossa structures, diminished rCBF was also considered if the isotope uptake count was 75% or lower in relation to the cerebellar area with the greatest uptake.

The patients' condition after the follow-up period was obtained from the hospital medical records and classified according to their clinical and SPECT status. For evaluating the results, these were classified as better, equal, or worse in respect to those of their initial assessment. Statistical analysis was performed by 2×2 tables, using the two-tailed Fischer exact test, and the results were considered statistically significant for a P value of .05 or lower.

On the other hand, a search of the current literature on SPECT scanning in ACs was performed by the PubMed database and the list was improved by manual search of the references found in the selected publications.

RESULTS OF SPECT STUDIES

Own Experience

The preliminary study [15] comprised 20 consecutive subjects whose cysts were distributed as follows: 11 in the sylvian fissure (Fig. 16.1), four in the posterior fossa, three at the midline (Fig. 16.2), and three within the lateral ventricles (Fig. 16.3). In six instances, the ACs were situated on the right hemisphere and four on the left. One patient had bilateral temporal cysts (Fig. 16.4). The subgroup of sylvian cysts consisted of 11 patients (six male and five female) with ages from 2 to 42 (median 12) years. Seven patients were 17 years of age or younger. At presentation, 10 patients were symptomatic and referred a diversity of complaints. One

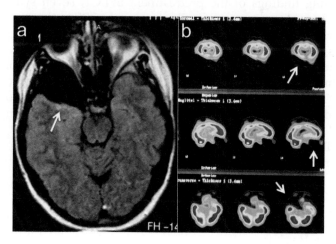

FIGURE 16.1   (A) MRI of a 9-year-old boy with a right sylvian arachnoid cyst (arrow). (B) Presurgical SPECT scan of the same patient in the coronal (upper row), sagittal (middle row), and axial plane (lower row) showing hypoperfusion close to the cyst (arrows).

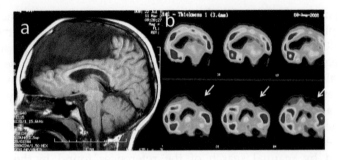

FIGURE 16.2   (A) MRI of a 10-year-old boy with severe headaches showing a frontal interhemispheric arachnoid cyst. (B) SPECT study depicting diminished uptake surrounding the cyst (arrows).

of the pediatric patients harbored bilateral incidental ACs that were disclosed during the routine clinical evaluation of neurofibromatosis type 1 (Fig. 16.4). Hydrocephalus was found in only one patient.

Skull radiographs showed signs of intracranial hypertension in three instances, skull asymmetry with cranial bulging in two, focal pressure signs in two, and dilated paranasal sinuses (pneumosinus dilatans) in two, being normal in two further cases. EEG showed focal or diffuse abnormalities in six instances and was normal in the remaining five cases. CT and/or MRI depicted the situation and size of the ACs and was also useful in demonstrating brain shifts, brain compression, and hydrocephalus. Most ACs (9 of 11) had a mean diameter larger than 3 cm, while in two this diameter was smaller than 3 cm.

Regarding findings of the pretreatment SPECT, seven symptomatic patients showed an image of focally decreased rCBF in the surrounding brain surface that was in close contact with the cyst's walls. Four other instances, including the asymptomatic patient, showed a normal SPECT scan. Four patients were given a cystoperitoneal (CP) derivation as initial treatment and two of them were given an additional ventriculoperitoneal (VP) shunt. Six patients were submitted to observation consisting of periodical clinical and neuroimaging assessment. Following treatment, all patients were again evaluated with a SPECT scan. At the end of the follow-up, rCBF in four operated and in one nonoperated patient had normalized and the patients were clinically improved. At the same time, the six subjects submitted to conservative treatment were clinically stable and had an unchanged SPECT.

Literature Review

In our literature search, we found several case reports on SPECT use in patients with ACs [17–21,23,24]. Holman et al. [16] elaborated a method of superimposition of magnetic resonance and high-resolution

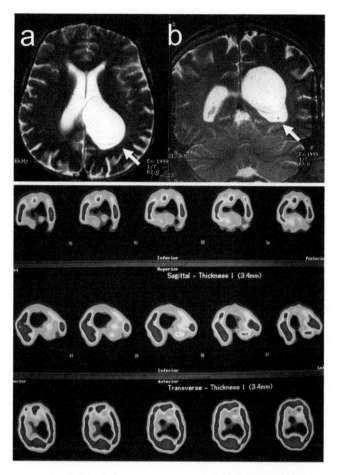

FIGURE 16.3 (A) Axial cuts of a MRI corresponding to an 18-year-old girl with incapacitating positional headaches and (B) coronal cuts showing a left intraventricular arachnoid cyst. Lower rows: SPECT scanning in coronal, sagittal and axial planes showing decreased perfusion in the brain areas surrounding the cyst.

Technetium-99m-HHMPAO and Thallium-201 SPECT images for studying patients with dementia or focal cerebral lesions, including one case with a right middle fossa AC, focal lesions observed on MRI corresponded well with areas of perfusion defects on SPECT [16]. On the contrary, SPECT results do not always corresponded with the epilepsy foci [18,19].

Other publications refer to short series of patients with ACs evaluated with SPECT scanning. Sgouros and Chapman [13] described zones of *diffuse hypoperfusion*, while Germano et al. [14] and Martínez-Lage et al. [15] reported a different pattern of impaired rCBF consisting of *focal* reduction in the zone surrounding the AC. Sato et al. [3] reported

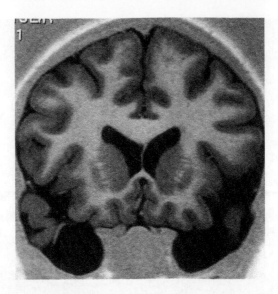

FIGURE 16.4   Coronal MRI cuts showing bilateral temporal arachnoid cysts in a young girl studied in the course of routine screening for neurofibromatosis type I.

an abnormal pattern of the rCBF that corresponded to larger cysts causing midline shifts and to those with hydrocephalus. Sato et al. also recommended surgery in infants as soon as possible to prevent irreversible brain damage.

DISCUSSION

Some considerations have to be taken into account from the start in this discussion [25]. (1) Most publications on the value of SPECT scanning (and of other functional studies) consist of samples of small size and with poorly controlled design. (2) There are no studies on cost–benefit of so-called functional studies. (3) Serious complications of surgery, such as hemorrhage, cerebral infarction, infections, and neurological deficits are hard to accept, which obliges the improvement of the indications for surgery. (4) The objective improvement after the diverse modalities of AC treatment is often difficult to validate and quantify.

Significance of Functional Studies for Deciding AC Surgery

Symptoms directly related with the presence of an AC are caused by local pressure, by displacement or distortion of neural structures, by intracranial hypertension, or by obstruction of CSF pathways. When the patients present with obvious symptoms and signs of cerebral dysfunction or of raised ICP, indications for surgical treatment are straightforward [1]. In infants, macrocephaly, skull asymmetry, or cranial bulging are often considered as indications for surgical treatment. Macrocephaly in neonates and infants with ACs usually means increased ICP due to associated hydrocephalus or to the presence of large or giant cysts, conditions that call for surgical treatment [3].

However, ACs may occur with more subtle clinical manifestations that eventually might favor surgical treatment [5–7]. These include headaches, dizziness, epilepsy (without a clear epileptogenic focus), developmental delay, and certain neurocognitive, behavioral, or psychiatric disorders, although some authors might think they may represent a fortuitous association. Among these vague symptoms, headaches and dizziness constitute the most common and unspecific complaints. These complaints might also be attributable to a variety of conditions. On assessing neurodevelopmental delay, the clinician is obliged to exclude beforehand other etiologies that might be responsible for it. Cognitive, behavioral, and psychiatric conditions, which are sometimes found in patients with ACs, require additional specialized studies, such as formal neuropsychological testing and consultation with a neuropsychologist [7].

Obviously, asymptomatic and incidental ACs, even those of large size, are best managed conservatively and often necessitate only periodic clinical and neuroimaging evaluation [26–28]. Some publications have shown that a mild increase in cyst size during follow-up has no pathological significance and does not indicate brain damage [22]. However, not all investigators agree with this view and prefer to adopt a more liberal attitude to not overlook the eventual production of a protracted neurological damage [5–7].

Isotope-Based Studies in the Assessment of AC Pathology

Several procedures that utilize isotopes have been utilized in the diagnostic assessment of ACS and are summarized in Table 16.1.

1. *Isotopic brain scan.* Prior to the introduction of CT and MRI in clinical practice, early reports on methods for AC diagnosis comprised isotopic brain scans. This study was rather unspecific and depicted only large lesions causing a significant brain damage [29]. These authors reported two patients suspected of having an AC. The first was a patient with decreased uptake in the sequential isotopic brain study that displayed a normal definitive brain scan. The other patient showed increased uptake in a sylvian AC that the authors attributed to an underlying subdural hematoma. Tuynman et al. [30] reported a

TABLE 16.1　Isotope Diagnostic Tools for Assessing Functional Anomalies in Intracranial ACs

Diagnostic tool	Indication/Use
Brain scan	Detection of mass effect
Isotope cisternography	Depiction of cyst communication with arachnoid spaces and cisterns
Isotopic shuntogram	Detection of shunt patency
PET	Depiction of brain metabolism anomalies
SPECT	Detection of changes in cerebral blood flow

child with bilateral temporal ACs, but only one of the cysts showed a local increase uptake of radiotracer that suggested a brain tumor but that was a cyst with thickened membranes probably due to a previous cyst hemorrhage. In the case documented by Yokoyama et al. [31] increased uptake of radiotracer was also attributed to a coexistent subdural hematoma.

2. *Isotopic cisternography.* Radioisotopic cisternography and ventriculography were introduced by Di Chiro et al. [32] for studying CSF circulation. In addition to conventional postcontrast cisternography, some investigators mainly utilized isotopic cisternography for assessing the eventual communication of the AC with the cisterns and subarachnoid spaces. This method also informed on the early and late behavior of the radiotracer communication and on its behavior in the surrounding brain parenchyma. Goluboff [33] reported one case of posterior fossa AC with midline increased isotope activity that showed communication and stressed its value in the differential diagnosis with other cystic lesions in this location. Handa et al. [34] demonstrated the existence of communication in two instances of ACs. Ferreira et al.'s [35] case showed this communication, which in their opinion supported conservative treatment. Seur and Kooman [36], also confirmed the existence of communication in their case together with a slow flow within the cyst. In rare cases of syringomyelia associated with intracranial ACs, isotopic cisternography may also show the site and extension of the syrinx In rare cases of syringomyelia associated with intracranial ACs, isotopic cisternography may also show the site and extension of the syrinx (Fig. 16.5).

3. *Radionuclide shuntography.* Some patients with intracranial ACs are given a CP or VP shunt. Devices for CSF drainage may be obstructed by a variety of causes. Shunt failure can present acutely with alarming signs of brain herniation and need emergent evaluation and

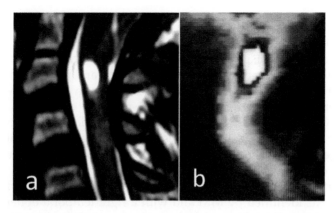

FIGURE 16.5 (A) MRI of a 12-year-old boy with a supratentorial arachnoid cyst showing tonsillar descent, syringomyelia, and spinal cord edema below the syrinx. (B) Isotopic cisternography showing increased radiotracer uptake probably indicating spinal cord damage.

treatment. More often shunt malfunction presents in subacute or chronic ways permitting a less stressful evaluation. Radionuclide CSF shunt testing can diagnose shunt patency and differentiate proximal from distal block. In addition, the exact place of CSF blockage can be demonstrated by showing where the isotope progression stops. The technique consists of the injection of 0.25—1.5 mCi of Tc-pertechnetate in the shunt reservoir, obtaining dynamic images (30 seconds per frame) for approximately 30 minutes [37]. Isotopic activity progresses along the shunt tubing and spreads out rapidly at the distal end of the drainage (usually the peritoneum).

4. *Positron emission tomography.* PET scans are utilized to detect malignancies, cerebrovascular disorders, sequels of brain trauma, hydrocephalus, postradiation necrosis versus recurrence, and exceptionally for assessing intracranial cystic lesions. De Volder et al. [11] reported a 10-year-old child with acquired childhood aphasia who harbored an AC on his left sylvian region. CT and MRI in this child failed to discover any mass effect on the surrounding brain. However, SPECT study showed pronounced hypometabolism around the cyst involving the speech areas. After CP shunting, a significant metabolic improvement was shown in the affected areas. Tripathi et al. [12] in a review paper, documented, the PET findings in a case of AC as a mass with slight distortion of adjacent brain structures without peripheral contrast enhancement, thus contributing to the differential diagnosis of hypometabolic-hypodense lesions on PET-TC. An interesting case of an incidental giant right frontal AC discovered during PET-TC screening for suspicion of mediastinal sarcoidosis was reported by Hubele et al. [10].

SPECT

This diagnostic method is habitually used for assessment of rCBF in different conditions, e.g., in head injury, dementia, cerebrovascular diseases, epilepsy, normal pressure hydrocephalus, and pseudotumor cerebri. Several anecdotal case reports of SPECT use in patients with ACs have been published. Henkes et al. [23] reported eight cases studied with SPECT and subsequent 3D rendering in addition to rectilinear CSF imaging in diverse clinical conditions. Scans generated 4–24 hours after tracer injection were superior in the delineation of basal cisterns, especially for detecting cystic lesions close to the cranial base [23].

Kuwert et al. [19] reported an interesting case of a patient with a left temporal AC identified by MRI and with a right temporal epileptogenic focus. In this patient hypoperfusion was found contralaterally to the MRI abnormality but ipsilaterally to the pathological EEG focus [19].

Urasaki et al. [21] documented a decrease of rCBF on the right hemisphere in the SPECT of a 17-year-old boy with a frontotemporal AC diagnosed with choreoathetosis. This patient also had right basal ganglia and adjacent area of increased activity in the frontal region [21]. The patient reported by Tsurushima et al. [20], studied by vertigo and behavior disturbances, had decreased rCBF in the left frontal region coinciding with an AC. The hypoperfusion reversed after craniotomy and cyst decompression.

Kidooka et al. [18] reported a child with agenesis of the internal carotid artery and a retrocerebellar AC studied with SPECT that ascertained no hypoperfusion area. Horiguchi and Takeshita [24] have also documented abnormal perfusion in a child with a left frontal fossa AC who presented with cognitive function and impaired language.

Kang et al. [17] presented a patient with behavioral problems studied by SPECT that showed a cystic image in the posterior fossa corresponding to a large mega cisterna magna and discussed its differential diagnosis of ACs with Dandy-Walker malformation. Holman et al. [16] developed a method of superimposition of magnetic resonance and high-resolution Technetium-99m-HHMPAO and Thallium-201 SPECT images and studied nine patients with dementia or focal cerebral lesions, including one case with a right middle fossa AC, and four normal controls. Focal lesions observed on MRI corresponded to areas of perfusion defects on SPECT [16].

Sgouros and Chapman [13] reported three children with ACs who were evaluated by SPECT scanning demonstrating *global hypoperfusion*. In the first, a 3-year-old boy with a middle fossa AC, the SPECT disclosed bilateral deep white matter defects of perfusion in the ipsilateral basal ganglia. The second one was a 17-year-old boy with a middle fossa AC that showed in his SPECT study significant perfusion defects in the deep white matter of both brain hemispheres close to the basal ganglia. In the third child, a 6-year-old boy diagnosed with a sylvian AC, the SPECT showed bilateral perfusion defects in the deep white matter of both parietal lobes. Interestingly, the areas of defective perfusion had a normal appearance in MRI studies. After surgical treatment, these perfusion completely disappeared. This was accompanied by general improvement of the preexisting nonspecific symptoms.

Germano et al. [14] documented two infants, aged 23 and 29 days respectively, with macrocrania, split sutures, and bulging fontanels. Both children had large fronto-temporo-parietal cysts and were treated with CP shunts using a programmable Hakim valve. In the two infants, SPECT disclosed *local* hypoperfusion zones in the areas surrounding the cysts. Surgical decompression led to normalization of the rCBF in both instances.

Martínez-Lage et al. [15] performed a study of 20 patients with ACs, 11 with middle fossa cysts, studied with SPECT scanning. Their main finding was to describe a *focal* reduction in cerebral perfusion in the zone surrounding the AC but no global cerebral perfusion defects. They also attested the value of cerebral SPECT as an adjunctive tool for detecting functional anomalies to allocate the patients for surgical or conservative management. SPECT in AC evaluation also is useful in differentiating active damage from focal brain atrophy in ACs [15]. In addition, SPECT scanning might also be of help in locating the cyst responsible for the patient's symptoms in cases with bilateral or multiple ACs.

Sato et al. [3] undertook a prospective study of 48 patients with middle fossa ACs, 18 of them being symptomatic. The study protocol comprised CT and/or MRI, quantitative CT-cisternography, digital angiography, IMP-SPECT, and psychomotor analysis. An abnormal pattern of the rCBF evaluated with I-IMP-SPECT was found in 11 (23%) of cases, which corresponded to larger cysts with midline shift and to those with hydrocephalus. This was a reversible low-perfusion pattern showing early low distribution and delayed redistribution. After craniotomy and membranectomy, the brain perfusion normalized. These authors attribute the abnormal rCBF to mild but chronic pressure on the veins. Sato et al. also recommend surgery in infants as soon as possible during the ontogenic period of rapid myelination when reversible brain growth is more likely.

CONCLUSIONS

There is much debate on which ACs actually produce neurological damage and on which ones should be treated with surgery or be simply observed. US, CT, and MRI constitute the habitual imaging studies that give information on ACS' morphological details. Anatomical features comprise cyst location and size, brain compression, shifts, and existence of hydrocephalus. From the current literature on the subject, it is obvious that functional studies devised to evaluate the neurological damage produced by the cysts in the patients are crucial for allocating them for surgical or conservative management. EEG, functional MRI, ICP monitoring, neuropsychological testing, and PET scanning are among the most utilized tests for assessing brain dysfunction caused by ACs. However, no single procedure has been shown to be capable of detecting the actual degree of brain damage produced by the cyst. In the authors' experience cerebral SPECT studies provide worthy information on rCBF changes produced by the ACs. Thus, in the appropriate clinical setting, cerebral SPECT constitutes a valuable adjunct tool for establishing the indications for surgery in patients diagnosed with ACs. As in many other neurosurgical conditions, presently the decision about undertaking surgical treatment should be based mainly on a solid clinical basis.

References

[1] Wilkinson CC, Winston KR. Congenital arachnoid cysts and Dandy-Walker complex. In: Albright AL, Pollack IF, Adelson PD, editors. Principles and practice of pediatric neurosurgery. 2nd ed. New York, Stuttgart: Thieme; 2008. p. 162–86.

[2] Galassi E, Piazza G, Gaist G, Frank F. Arachnoid cysts of the middle cranial fossa: a clinical and radiological study of 25 cases treated surgically. Surg Neurol 1980;14:211–19.

[3] Sato H, Sato N, Katayama S, Tamaki N, Matsumoto S. Effective shunt-independent treatment for primary middle fossa arachnoid cyst. Childs Nerv Syst 1991;7:375–81.

[4] Martínez-Lage JF, Pérez-Espejo MA, Almagro MJ, López López-Guerrero A. Hydrocephalus and arachnoid cysts. Childs Nerv Syst 2011;27:1643–52.

[5] Helland AC, Wester K. A population-based study of intracranial arachnoid cysts: clinical and neuroimaging studies following surgical cyst decompression in children. J Neurosurg 2006;105(Suppl 5):385–90.

[6] Helland AC, Wester K. A population-based study of intracranial arachnoid cysts: clinical and neuroimaging studies following surgical cyst decompression in adults. J Neurol Neurosurg Psychiatry 2007;78:1129–35.

[7] Gjerde PB, Schmid M, Hammar Ä, Wester K. Intracranial arachnoid cysts: impairment of higher cognitive functions and postoperative improvement. J Neurodev Dis 2013;5:21.

[8] Di Rocco C, Tamburrini G, Caldarelli M, Velardi F, Santini P. Prolonged ICP monitoring in Sylvian arachnoid cysts. Surg Neurol 2003;60:211–18.

[9] Paetau R, Kajola M, Karhu J, Nousiainen U, Partanen J, Tihonen J, et al. Magnetoencephalographic localization of epileptic cortex—impact on surgical treatment. Ann Neurol 1992;32:106–9.

[10] Hubele F, Imperiale A, Kremer S, Namer IJ. Asymptomatic giant arachnoid cyst. Clin Nucl Med 2012;37:982–3.

[11] De Volder AG, Michel Cl, Thauvoy C, Willems G, Ferrièr G. Brain glucose utilization in acquired childhood aphasia associated with a sylvian arachnoid cyst: recovery after shunting as demonstrated by PET. J Neurol Neurosurg Psychiatry 1994;57: 296−300.

[12] Tripathi M, Jaimini A, D'Souza MM, Sharma R, Jain J, Garg G, et al. Spectrum of brain abnormalities detected on whole body F-18 FDG PET/TC in patients undergoing evaluation for non-CNS malignancies. Indian J Nucl Med 2011;26:123−9.

[13] Sgouros S, Chapman SS. Congenital middle fossa arachnoid cysts may cause global brain ischaemia: a study with ^{99}TC-hexamethylpropylene-amineoxime single photon emission computerized tomography scans. Pediatr Neurosurg 2001;35:188−94.

[14] Germano A, Caruso G, Caffo M, Baldari S, Calisto A, Meli F, et al. The treatment of large supratentorial arachnoid cysts in infants with cyst-peritoneal shunting and Hakim programmable valve. Childs Nerv Syst 2003;19:166−73.

[15] Martínez-Lage JF, Valentí JA, Piqueras C, Ruiz-Espejo AM, Román F, Nuño de la Rosa JA. Functional assessment of intracranial arachnoid cysts with TC99 m-HMPAO SPECT: a preliminary report. Childs Nerv Syst 2006;22:1091−7.

[16] Holman BH, Zimmerman RE, Johnson KA, Carvalho PA, Schwartz RB, Loeffler JS, et al. Computer-assisted superimposition of magnetic resonance and high-resolution Technetium-99m-HMPAO and Thallium-201 SPECT images of the brain. J Nucl Med 1991;32:1478−84.

[17] Kang PS, Caride VJ. Functional brain imaging in a patient with giant cisterna Magna. Clin Nucl Med 2002;27:827−38.

[18] Kidooka M, Okada T, Handa J. Agenesis of the internal carotid artery − report of a case combined with arachnoid cyst in a child. No Shinkei 1992;44:371−5 (Japanese).

[19] Kuwert T, Stodieck SR, Puskás C, Diehl B, Puskás Z, Schuierer G, et al. Reduced GABAA receptor density contralateral to a potentially epileptogenic MRI abnormality in a patient with complex partial seizures. Eur J Nucl Med 1996;23:95−8.

[20] Tsurushima H, Harakuni T, Saito A, Tominaga D, Hyodo A, Yoshii Y. Symptomatic arachnoid cyst of the left frontal convexity presenting with memory disturbance. Neurol Med Chir (Tokyo) 2000;40:339−41.

[21] Urasaki E, Tokimura T, Genmoto T, Yokota A. Paroxysmal kinesigenic choreoathetosis associated with frontotemporal arachnoid cyst. Case report. Neurol Med Chir (Tokyo) 1999;39:169−73.

[22] Shim KW, Lee YH, Park EK, Park YS, Choi JU, Kim DS. Treatment option for arachnoid cysts. Childs Nerv Syst 2009;25:1459−66.

[23] Henkes H, Huber G, Hierholzer J, Cordes M, Kujat C, Piepgras U. Radionuklidzisternographie: SPECT und 3D-Tecchnik. Radiologe 1991;31:489−95.

[24] Horiguchi T, Takeshita K. Cognitive function and language in a child with an arachnoid cyst in the left frontal fossa. World J Biol Psychiatry 2000;1:159−63.

[25] Rabiei K, Högfeldt MJ, Doria-Medina R, Tisell M. Surgery for intracranial arachnoid cysts in children −a prospective long-term study. Childs Nerv Syst 2016;32:1257−63.

[26] Aoki N, Sakai T, Umezawa Y. Slit ventricle syndrome after cyst-peritoneal shunting for the treatment of intracranial arachnoid cyst. Childs Nerv Syst 1990;6:41−3.

[27] Martínez-Lage JF, Ruíz-Espejo AM, Almagro MJ, Alfaro R, Felipe-Murcia M, López López-Guerrero A. CSF overdrainage in shunted intracranial arachnoid cysts: a series and review. Childs Nerv Syst 2009;25:1061−9.

[28] Di Rocco C. Sylvian fissure arachnoid cysts: we do operate on them but should it be done? Childs Nerv Syst 2010;26:173−5.

[29] Weinberg PE, Flom RA. Intracranial subarachnoid cysts. Radiology 1973;106:329−33.

[30] Tuynman FHB, Hekster REM, Pauwels EKJ. Intracranial arachnoid cyst of the middle fossa demonstrated by positive 99m TC brainscintigraphy. Neuroradiology 1973;7: 41−4.

[31] Yokoyama K, Tonami N, Kimura M, Kinoshita A, Aburano T, Hisada K. Scintigraphic demonstration of intracranial communication between arachnoid cyst and associated subdural hematoma. Clin Nucl Med 1989;14:350–3.
[32] Di Chiro G, Reames PM, Matthews WB. Risa-ventriculography and risa-cisternography. Neurology 1964;14:185–91.
[33] Goluboff LG. Arachnoid cyst of the posterior fossa demonstrated by isotope cisternography. J Nucl Med 1973;14:61–2.
[34] Handa J, Nakano Y, Aii H. CT cisternography with intracranial arachnoid cysts. Surg Neurol 1977;8:451–4.
[35] Ferreira S, Jhingran SG, Johnson PC. Radionuclide cisternography in the study of arachnoid cysts. Neuroradiology 1980;19:167–9.
[36] Seur NH, Kooman A. Arachnoid cyst of the middle cranial fossa with paradoxical changes of the bony structures. Neuroradiology 1976;12:177–83.
[37] Goeser CD, McLeary MS, Young LW. Diagnostic imaging of ventriculoperitoneal shunt malfunctions and complications. Radiographics 1998;18:635–51.

Index

Printed and bound by CPI Group (UK) Ltd, Croydon, CR0 4YY

03/10/2024

01040420-0004